Soccer Functional Fitness Training

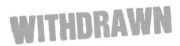

The contents of this book were carefully researched. However, all information is supplied without liability. Neither the author nor the publisher will be liable for possible disadvantages or damages resulting from this book.

DOST, TE POEL, HYBALLA

SOCCER
FUNCTIONAL
FITNESS TRAINING

Meyer & Meyer Sport

Original title: Fußballfitness - Athletiktraining, Meyer & Meyer Verlag Aachen, 2015
Translation: AAA Translation, St. Louis, Missouri

British Library Cataloguing in Publication Data
A catalogue record for this book is available from the British Library

Soccer Functional Fitness Training
Maidenhead: Meyer & Meyer Sport (UK) Ltd., 2016
ISBN: 978-1-78255-090-7

© 2016 by Meyer & Meyer Sport (UK) Ltd.
Aachen, Auckland, Beirut, Cairo, Cape Town, Dubai, Hägendorf, Hong Kong,
Indianapolis, Manila, New Delhi, Singapore, Sydney, Tehran, Vienna
Member of the World Sport Publishers' Association (WSPA)
Manufacturing by: Print Consult, Munich
ISBN: 978-1-78255-090-7
E-Mail: info@m-m-sports.com
www.m-m-sports.com

CONTENTS

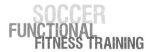

ACKNOWLEDGMENTS

A huge thank-you to the many coaches and especially the experts Hans Meyer, Fred Rutten, and Erik ten Hag (all with FC Twente). Their needs and many questions helped me optimize the fitness requirements of the players entrusted to me in terms of professional soccer. The teamwork with Hans-Dieter and Peter was more than excellent. Harteliijk, thank you!

—Harry Dost

I would like to dedicate this book particularly to my supporters and companions Dr. J. Eulering (North Rhine-Westphalia/LSBNRW), Dr. K. Paul (Hesse), Dr. R. Naul (Essen-Duisburg/Münster), Dr. A. Neumaier (DSHS Cologne/Bochum), Dr. W. Kuhn (DSHS Cologne/Berlin), Dr. D. Teipel (DHS Cologne/Jena), Dr. St. Starischka (Dortmund), Dr. M. Grosser (Munich), R. Fuchs (Munich), Paul Wagner (Olympic base camp Rhein-Ruhr), R. Herings (1.FC Cologne), K.H. Drygalsky (Borussia Mönchengladbach), the colleagues at the state training centers in Straelen and Essen and the national training center in Dortmund, former coaches, all of the German-Dutch coaches, and the German Sports University Cologne. A heartfelt thank-you to my friends and superb experts and human beings: my colleagues Harry, Peter, and Eduard. The teamwork was simply outstanding: "Here is to an even better (human) sport!"

—Hans-Dieter te Poel

I dedicate this book to all German-Dutch soccer coaches, and a great big thank-you to my two top-coaching colleagues, Hans-Dieter and Harry, for the awesome and interesting collaboration!

–Peter Hyballa

www.peterhyballa.org

Assisted by Eduard Feldbusch

(Sport and Performance Science major at the German Sports University Cologne; eduard@feldbusch-cat.de)

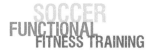

PREFACE

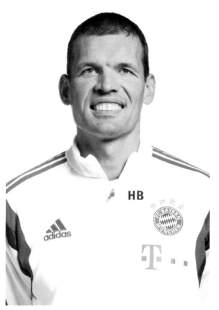

HB

Many textbooks have been written about soccer. It is common knowledge that the game has changed tremendously in recent decades. It has become faster;tackling has become tougher; and physical demands have increased significantly. This also brings into question the traditional schools of thought.

When should youth training begin, and what should an approach that is developmental, sports-scientific, and soccer-specific look like? This book tries to provide answers to these questions.

In doing so, the authors place special emphasis on the coupling of existing textbook knowledge and current international research literature that is based on soccer-specific issues. Nowadays, it is no longer enough to advocate the age-old soccer wisdoms of "it matters on the field" or "the round must go into the square."

Anyone expecting "recipes" in this book will be disappointed. That expectation is unrealistic at a time when the peak of performance in soccer, too, is determined by the top 3 to 5% of all fitness-related, technical–tactical, and mental abilities.

On the contrary, today, and in the future, an active, interested, and engaged reader with known and solid findings in the light of new scientific research results is absolutely essential.

This book offers a very good foundation.

I hope all of the readers will not only enjoy reading this book, but also feel motivated to try out and further develop its suggestions.

–Dr. Holger Broich
Director of Health and Fitness, FC Bayern Munich
Munich, Germany, March 2015

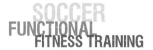
INTRODUCTION

"Yes. There are more objectives after winning the title, whereby I have always evaluated my work and myself independent of any titles. ...How is world soccer evolving and where do we want to be in 2016? How do we want our team to play?"

(DFB national team coach, Joachim Löw, quoted in kicker, 104, p. 13, December 22, 2014)

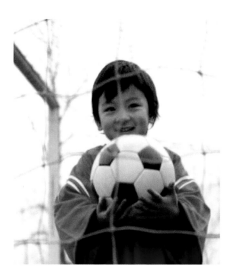

Young soccer players, coaches, and instructors often ask when they should introduce physical training in their soccer instruction, how to integrate fitness or athletic training into soccer training, and which types of drills and games to use as a basis for training. Due to frequently limited training volume yet high competitive workload and demands, particularly in amateur soccer, there is the additional issue of planned and organized fitness or athletic training usually not starting until players have moved up to the men's or women's leagues. In addition, with the start of puberty, ambitious youth and men and women players often do individual at home or fitness facility training that is rarely coordinated or discussed with the team coach with respect to content and methodology. Often well-intended individual measures result in a conglomeration of training loads that are, in part, contrary to the intentions of modern soccer training and have not been correlated with a soccer player's demand profile.

Building too much muscle mass accompanied by decreased flexibility (also in the area of technical motor skills), decreased endurance, and higher frequency of injuries are just a few of the ascertainable negative side effects.

When asked about the previous topics, the authors always issue the following statement:

Physical training begins with youth players, and training of fitness-related performance factors in soccer differs from adult training in quantity and quality.

But what is physical training in the sense of modern fitness or athletic training in soccer?

The subject discipline generally defines a player's physical performance capacity as the fitness-related performance factors **endurance, strength, speed,** and **agility** (Weineck, 2004, p. 11). Since agility is not only correlative to endurance ability, but also impacts particularly coordination and technique (here with respect to an optimally dynamic spatial–temporal execution), the authors will also address optimal coordination training in soccer in subsequent chapters (see chapters 3, 4, and 17; compare Weineck, Memmert, and Uhin, 2012). We, thereby, also follow the current curricula and study regulations for the sports discipline, which is giving the area of coordination and technique increasingly more room for theoretical contemplation and practical implementation during classes and in courses.

The authors chose a structure that applies to the well-known image of the hardware store, i.e. the reader may arrange his materials as required for his team. He has free choice. Since there is no general theory for soccer functional fitness training, at some points the authors deliberately offer theoretical set pieces to the reader. However, those were all carefully researched from primary sources from Germany and abroad and highlighted in the text passages concerned. In this way, our standards for scientific work shall be maintained in the whole book.

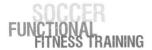
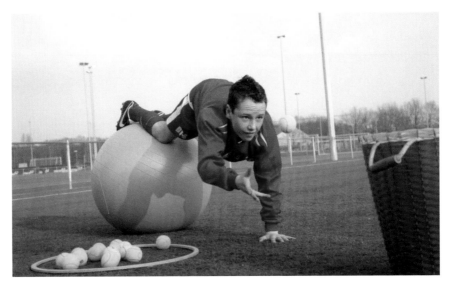

Photo 1: Game-like development of trunk stability

Because, without an adequately developed coordinationfoundation, we soccer players have trouble with the ball. We want to be boss on the ball!

Furthermore, in this book, the authors focus on the *basicforms of movement*, the *skills*. This generally includes instruction in athletic movement in the form of running, skipping, and throwing (compare chapters 9-15). Elements of strength training that are completed in almost game-like form on the practice field are covered in chapter 16.

Once soccer performance increases during training and in competition, more specific training methods are introduced more frequently to raise the soccer player's performance level. Because, in general, top soccer players like Cristiano Ronaldo are characterized by their extremely high athletic performance capacity. That is why *general* and *specific strength training* (with a view to elite soccer) takes on an important role in soccer instruction overall.

Some authors differentiate between the terms strength training and athletic training (Wirth et al., 2012, p. 33-39). When following this differentiation, and the authors wish to do so here, general strength training with medium and high loading intensities targets the development of maximum and explosive strength in the weight room. Athletic training uses a number of drills and types of games for the purpose of developing high-quality jumps, throws, and sprints. This is meant to help facilitate the transfer of the increased strength to the target movements in soccer (compare to Wirth et al., 2012, p. 39).

Therefore, athletic training should occupy a *hinge function* between strength abilities and target movements by means of quick movements and low resistance at the highest technical level.[1] It is geared toward the adequate adaptation of the player's functional system and follows the specific adaptation to imposed demand principle, also referred to as SAID principle, which, from a biological and sports scientific perspective, is beyond dispute (compare in particular Gambetta, 2007; Steinhöfer, 2008; and Issurin, 2013).

To continue to captivate youth players during long-term performance *development* strength training, in particular, that does not have a playful character and in the mid- and long-term requires a high degree of behavior control by all involved and should be constantly modified, presented, and implemented in an attractive manner. This presupposes creativity and inventiveness from coaches and instructors. This book is meant to inspire the same—a matter of great concern to the authors. The theoretical reference framework is chosen and presented in such a way as to refer to already existing findings using literary references. The authors hereby make room for the detailed, precise, and pictorial representation of the content of individual chapters that can then be put intopractice individually, group, and teamspecifically on the practice field. The authors provide additional suggestions for in-depth analyses and interpretation through corresponding literary references (see the references).

Anyone who works on his physical deficiencies without overdoing it will become a better player. The chain is as strong as its weakest link! However, this trite insight elucidates that a soccer player's weaknesses will surface, at the latest during competition. In chapters 9 through 20, the reader can find specific suggestions on how to eliminate them. At the same time, these practical suggestions are not

---

1   *The reader should consider this differentiation hereafter. Nevertheless, in training practice, the term strength training generally subsists so that, due to this lack of clarity, the authors subsequently refer to strength and athletic training.*

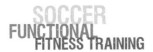
"recipes." Coaches, instructors, and players should always consider their institutional parameters, didactic and methodological prior knowledge, athletic objectives, and, especially in youth soccer, their social and educational intentions and use the presented drills and types of play accordingly.

> *"That is why I do a lot outside of practice as well. I go to the weight room or stay on the field longer. Players are getting younger and fitter. In the past we could solve problems visually. That is no longer possible today. To keep up at this high level you have to train intensively. But I feel good doing it."*

(Nelson Valdez, age 31, forward at Eintracht Frankfurt, in a kicker interview from February 23, 2015, 18, p. 78)

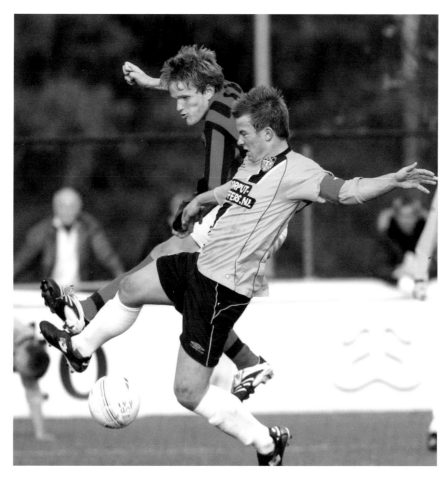

Photo 2: Absolute concentration in the battle for the ball

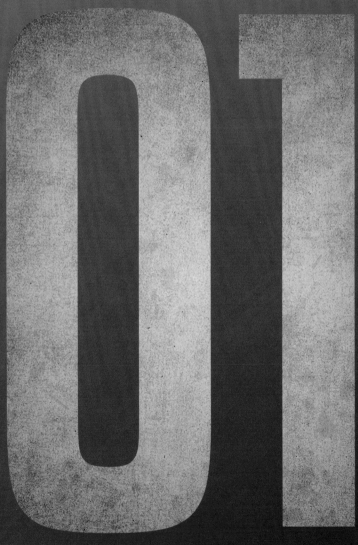

> CHAPTER

01

1 VERSALITY AS THE FOUNDATION FOR AN ASPIRING TOP SOCCER PLAYER

Germany is the 2014 World Champion:

"Mario Götze directs the rather horizontal trajectory of the ball forward into his running path with his slightly to the left facing chest, and after an intuitive right-left-right combination and a long step he slams the ball into the far corner with a left kick off the laces, next to the inside of the post, with centimeter precision."

(Karlheinz Wild, in kicker, November 3, 2014, 90, p. 8)

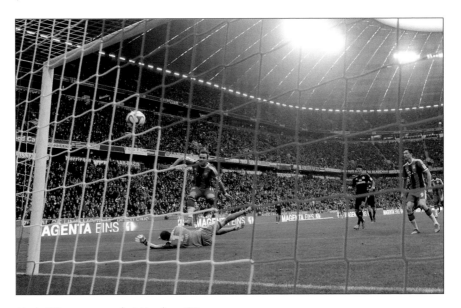

Mario Götze scores against Hamburg SV

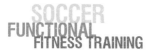

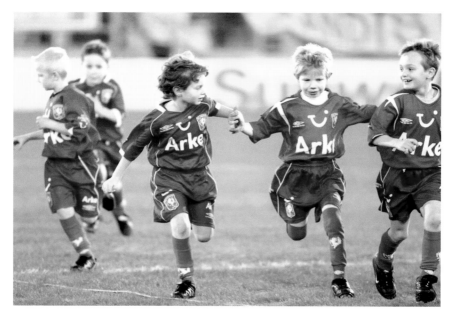

Photo 3: Friends playing together

Working *versatilely* with potential future top soccer players, especially in general and special instruction, is in many ways fascinating to dedicated coaches and instructors. Versatile people, in this case the coaches, instructors, and players, are open to just about anything and often impress their fellow human beings with their ability to effectively perceive and judge a situation, their ability to adapt to a situation appropriately and to quickly read a situation, and to act unexpectedly.

Addressing, refining, and developing these performance requirements in soccer to an individual's optimal potential represents a major challenge for the authors.

The awareness of this great responsibility plays an important role in today's modern soccer, which in recent years has rapidly evolved, particularly in the main areas of motor fitness: speed, coordination, strength, and endurance, even using different terminology:

"Soccer is a team sport, but in effect one must train like an individual sport. Tactics, technique, everything that happens on the field, happens within a team framework, but anything that happens before and after with respect to endurance, strength, speed, flexibility should be structured as individually as possible. Of course that is a major effort."

(Broich, July 8, 2013)[2]

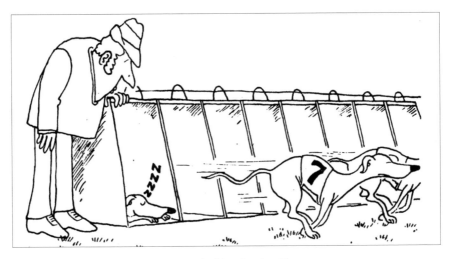

Fig. 1: Should the coach and instructor wake "sleeping dogs?"

In this context the term **versatility** represents a performance component to be accessed that is substantiated in professional literature as follows:

- Correspondence to the natural *movement requirements of* children and adolescents.
- *Requirements training* as basic conceptual orientation in the sense of presence of multidimensional plasticity. For example, versatility also means optimal development of jumping and rotational movements (left/right), often combined with spatial orientation.

2   *Holger Broich is a sports scientist at the German Sports University in Cologne, Germany, DFB U19 coach, athletic trainer, and was the fitness expert for Bayer 04 Leverkusen for 11 years. Since July 2014, he has been the performance diagnostician and fitness director for the reigning German champions FC Bayern Munich and, thereby, interfaces between Coach Pep Guardiola and the team physician, Dr. Hans-Wilhelm Müller-Wohlfahrt.*

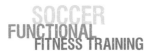
- ❂ Development and maintenance of *muscle balance* (prevention of muscular imbalance).
- ❂ *Prevention of structural uniformity* of training content and thereby premature and unintentional stagnation of performance development (particularly in advanced and high-performance training; see Martin et al., 1999, p. 253-259).
- ❂ Creating a *foundation of motor skills* to facilitate top performances in soccer.

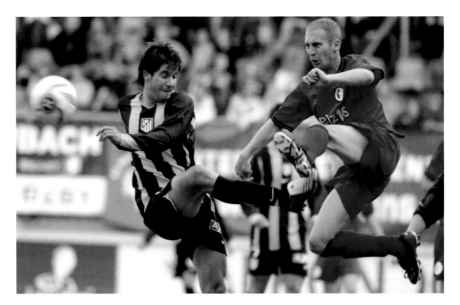

Photo 4: Controlling the ball while "floating" in the air and tackling without injuring each other [3]

Unfamiliar movement situations are resolved quicker and easier with a large repertoire of movements at one's disposal (i.e., wealth of movements and movement experience). Even with increasing age, a versatile training process is always linked to the growing specialization process and should prevent players from *specializing* too soon and too narrowly in soccer.

---

3   At times this is like figuring out $\sqrt{37597}$ and under lots of pressure of time and precision. The answer is training—extensive, intensive, and controlled training. This requires an expert. Without specific knowledge about functional relationships within the complex structure of soccer, objectives with, at times, major temporal and material effort are not adequately met. And quick repetition of a calculation on a calculator is, on the one hand, the arduous and lengthy catch-up on an absent player or, on the other hand, the correcting of ineffective fitness and athletic training. Without experts the entire training process can turn into an unpredictable risk for all involved.

But in the authors' opinion, **versatility** does not stand for randomness, aimlessness, and moving for the sake of moving. On the contrary, ambitious coaches and instructors usually pay attention to the structure of loading and stress and the desired effective direction when they choose drills and types of play and principles. In this book, *versatile training* focuses on the structure of the projected objective of the competitive activity in soccer (Martin et al. 1999) and today's developmental soccer instruction increasingly includes coordination abilities and skills, flexibility, strength, movement speed, and playing soccer.

Coordination training, under special consideration of empirical findings, should no longer be viewed and analyzed as conceptually separate from contemporary technical training in soccer (Hossner, 1995; Roth, 1996; Szymanski, 1997; Roth &Kröger, 2011; Weineck, Memmert and Uhing, 2012, p. 15).

This book shall contribute to expanding the individual's *versatility potential,* particularly in youth players, through a "large supply" of easily and quickly implemented drills and types of play. The variety of chosen training content and implementation procedures represent an important factor in athletic training – the subject of this book—because that is how versatile training of the central nervous system in particular becomes effective. Increasing maximum and explosive strength through, for instance, training with free weights will not be addressed hereafter. That would be the primary goal of "classic" weight training (Zawieja, 2008; Zawieja and Oltmanns, 2011).

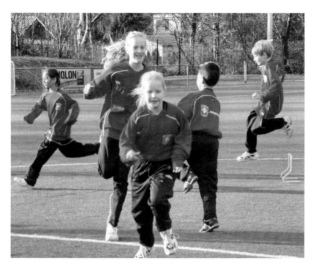

Photo 5: Discovering movement. Training can also be game-like.

> CHAPTER

02

2 FROM 0 TO 60! CREATING FOUNDATIONS TO GET TO THE TOP

> *"Games are won by athletes who concentrate on the playing field, not by those whose eyes are glued to the scoreboard."*

By now, it is a well-founded sports-scientific finding that a soccer player's athletic performance is determined by many coordinated, technical, psychosocial, physical fitness, mental, tactical cognitive, constitutional, and health-related factors (Weineck, 2004, p. 7; Weineck, 2007; see fig. 2).

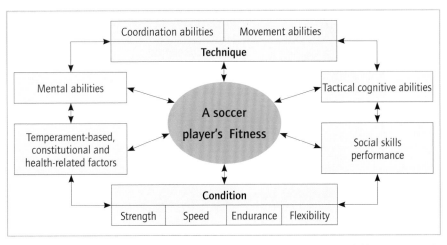

Fig. 2: The components of a soccer player's performance (Weineck, Memmert, and Uhing, 2012, p. 14)

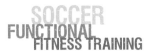

When taking additional current research results (Di Salvo et al., 2007, p. 224; Patra, 2011, p. 70) as a basis for the demand profile in today's elite soccer, it can be said with Weineck, Memmert, and Uhing (2012) that the coordinated, technical performance ability can be performance-limiting during the decisive phases of a competitive game "with the highest demands on acceleration/velocity and ball control" (p. 15).

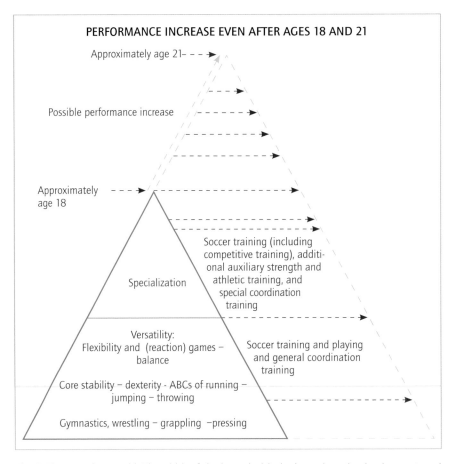

PERFORMANCE INCREASE EVEN AFTER AGES 18 AND 21

Approximately age 21-

Possible performance increase

Approximately age 18

Specialization

Soccer training (including competitive training), additional auxiliary strength and athletic training, and special coordination training

Versatility:
Flexibility and (reaction) games – balance

Soccer training and playing and general coordination training

Core stability – dexterity - ABCs of running – jumping – throwing

Gymnastics, wrestling – grappling –pressing

Fig. 3: The growth pyramid. The width of the base decisively determines the development goal or level.[4]

---

4   *The authors consider coordination training generally and specifically as coordinated supplementary training that serves the development of coordinated technical performance ability.*

Furthermore, the fitness-related demands on a professional soccer player are characterized by running distances of approximately 5.5 to 9 miles (depending on player and playing position) during a 90-minute game at a high "world competitive playing level" and hundreds of accelerations, jumps, passes, shots, headers, dribbles, and tackles. The fitness-related abilities determine a soccer player's performance ability as they represent the physical foundation of the complex ability to act (Weineck, Memmert, and Uhing, 2012, p. 14).

Accordingly, soccer training must build a *broad foundation* so that upcoming youth players are prepared for the enormous coordinated technical, fitness-related, and mental and intellectual demands and stress parameters and are able to still meet their individual performance potential after ages 18 and 21 through further performance increases by appropriate training. Figure 3 visualizes and substantiates this fundamental goal using the *growth pyramid.*

Figure 3 shows that the breadth of the foundation, meaning all presently known components of a soccer player's performance ability (Weineck, Memmert, and Uhing, 2012, p. 27; see fig. 2), determines the developmental goal and benefits a player's ability to *meet his individual performance potential* (goal is to reach top playing level) so that premature performance stagnation and barriers can be avoided.Also performance dips caused by physical and mental development spurts or environmental factors can be negotiated responsibly and appropriately for performance.[5]

Taking a look at, for instance, the training of young children (ages 7 to 13), we can see that emphasizing coordinated technical abilities promotes especially cognitive abilities, information processing, attention span, and playful creativity. Moreover, children achieve 80% of their permanent coordinated performance level by the end of elementary school age. Thus, it can be considered empirically substantiated that well-trained coordination abilities have an extremely positive effect on learning new things, their quality and variable and situational availability (Roth and Kröger, 2011).

---

5   *Beginning with the 2014/2015 season, Bundesliga clubs were able to freely decide whether to keep or eliminate their U23 teams. Some Bundesliga teams decided to release their coaches and players. The debate about the pros and cons of these decisions with respect to the quality of the training process has only just begun and should be closely monitored, primarily with regard to the development of youth players into pro soccer players by coaches and instructors.*

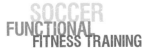

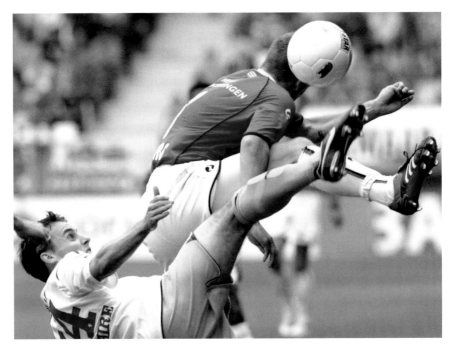

Photo 6: As a pro, assessing risk and showing courage is one thing...

As coaches and instructors, when working with children and adolescents, the authors have experienced that premature soccer training often results in talented children remaining "perpetual talents." Most of the time, they lack the *sport motor skill foundation while* developing their performance as a soccer player (see fig. 3) to be able to reach the top level. In addition, the frequently detected narrow foundation often results in stress intolerance and with increasing soccer-specific training volume and intensity, in *motivational problems and premature performance barriers or academic difficulties*, as well as *psychological problems* (te Poel & Hyballa, 2011).

The *growth pyramid* is also symbolic of the often not considered empirical fact that in today's soccer it can be assumed that trainability of, for instance, technical optimization is possible between the ages of 10 and 59, and the rate of learning can be seen as consistent (Wollny, 2002). According to this, one learns far beyond one's soccer career. The more motor skills one has "in the bag," the better, quicker, more precisely, variably, and economically one approaches the individual goal, the individual top performance level.

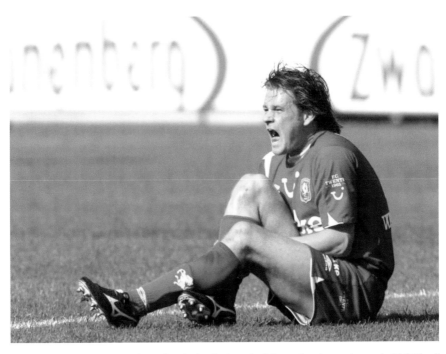

Photo 7: ...and tolerating pain and enduring is the other! Does the player give up inside? It's all about the attitude toward the game!

The *golden age* of learning in youth soccer does not exist because training spans the entire playing career; see *the growth pyramid* (Roth, 2005, p. 339).

A broad foundation, particularly with fitness-related and coordinated technical abilities, is a requirement for a soccer player to achieve his absolute performance ability.

The question of talent diagnostics is not discussed here because there has been much published on this topic in the past already (see Williams, Lee,and Reilly, 2000; Hohmann, 2001; Memmert and Roth, 2003; Neumann, 2009; Hyballa and te Poel, 2013). Instead, the authors will bring up a term here that plays an increasingly bigger role in today's instruction of pro soccer players in training and competition: **mindset.**

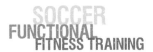

To the authors, **mindset** is a way of thinking about the pressure components, which include the following:

- *Playing for a big club and a select team and their implicit and explicit demands*
- One's own performance requirements
- Solving developmental tasks[6]
- The double stress and burden of competitive sport and school, college, job training, or profession
- The often high training intensity and volume
- The many competitions and routines
- The increasing rivalry between top teams
- The unforeseen behavior of opponents and teammates (e.g., during derby games and hard tackles;see chapter 16.3)
- Dealing with pain, injuries, and rehab
- Dealing with wins and losses
- The amount of travel and constantly changing accommodations
- Press reports and media coverage
- Expectations of parents, relatives, partners, and friends
- Difficult field and climate conditions

The soccer player should meet these head-on—anticipate them, recognize them, analyze them, and process them with attentiveness and concentration, emotional control, and frustration tolerance in a manner that benefits play and behavior. Because many a talent with aspirations of becoming a pro soccer player has foundered under these pressure components.

---

6   *Based on the developmental tasks concept, each person must solve certain developmental tasks during different phases of life. In youth competitive sports these are normative (e.g., acquiring a value system) and sport-related (e.g., learning emotional control) developmental tasks (Ohlert and Kleinert, 2014, p. 161-172).*

"There is no better recipe in soccer than work and faith in oneself. This combination will open any door. Everywhere. Kids need to internalize this. Of course there are players who possess fantastic skills, but they, too, have to work. You just don't see it. And sometimes there are younger players who don't get it. They think you either have it, or you don't. Wrong! You have to prove yourself everyday, even at practice. To the coach, the teammates, but most of all to yourself."

(FC Bayern Munich and Brazilian national team player Dante in a kicker interview with M. Zitouni, December 2, 2013, p. 13)

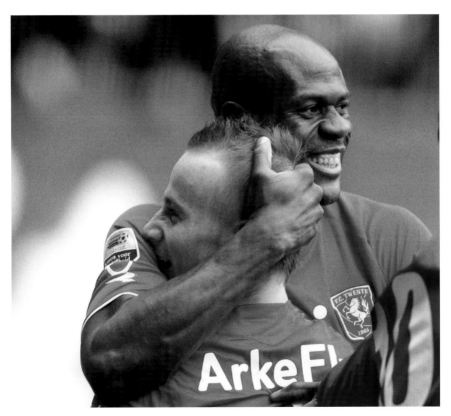

Photo 8: The joy over a mutual win outshines everything, especially when you have experienced the low points.

> CHAPTER

03

3 WHAT ARE COORDINATION ABILITIES AND VERSATILITY IN SOCCER?

The components of coordination abilities have been sufficiently addressed and at this point will be only briefly outlined within the context of their soccer-specific importance (for in-depth comparison, see Weineck, Memmert, and Uhing, 2012, p. 17-29):

- **Spatial and temporal orientation:** Sitting players in the space and quickly reading current and upcoming game situations (e.g., plays).

- The differentiation of movement sense (**differentiation ability**): Finely-tuned and controlled (timed) movements and partial body movements to be able to, for instance, use the arms situationally during a game tackle in a way that makes it possible to see the teammate or opponent and the ball at the same time and to achieve and retain the control to pass, dribble, or shoot. In soccer this is usually linked with orientation.

- Dynamic sense of balance (**balance ability**): Being able to quickly decelerate, twist, and turn without losing balance is a prerequisite for quick actions, especially in game situations. For beginners, but also for advanced players, jumping, fisting, heading, and throw-ins also require a well-developed dynamic sense of balance. In addition, when combined with technical training, it is possible to achieve sizeable progress in the coordinated technical optimization process. In youth and high-performance soccer, balance training is done specifically using game-specific drills and emphasized proprioceptive training.

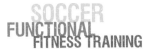

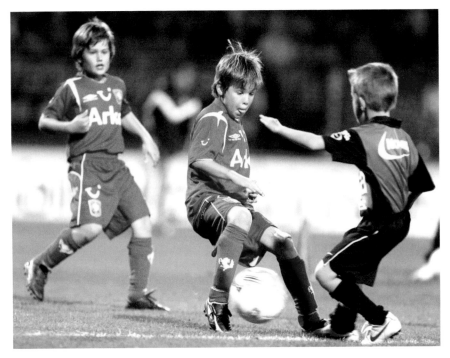

Photo 9: Dynamic sense of balance, keeping balance, and avoiding physical contac.

- Motor reaction—acoustic, tactile, and visual (**reaction ability**): The ability to quickly react to a signal with an appropriate motor action (e.g., a situation) is extremely important in soccer. Moreover, reaction ability is a subcomponent of the fitness skill **speed.**

- Sense of rhythm and tempo during complex movement structures (**ability to adjust and be rhythmic**): Being able to adjust movement while performing an action (e.g., slowing down or accelerating) or even changing it completely (e.g., switching the playing foot) is very important in soccer. Constantly adapting to the opponent and his playing style (e.g., changing system of play, type of pressing), external conditions (e.g., ground and climate conditions), and adjusting individual behaviors during different game scores and standings are important parts of the competitive game of soccer and require the appropriate practice and training. The individual dispositions of players must be taken into consideration during the training process: Am I a sensitive (passing) player who likes to play with the ball and its movement speed, or am I a more agile and fast player who often performs directional changes on the field with and without the ball?

❯ The ability to link motor movements **(linking ability):** Soccer techniques should be viewed as whole-body techniques. The ability to convert partial-body movements into an effective movement sequence during a target-oriented header requires early, intensive, and long-term practice and training (e.g., by means of Coerver Coaching).

But what the coordination ability components can accomplish in a soccer player's training process and which factors they are affected by are key issues in soccer practice and training.

COORDINATION ABILITIES

❯ are the basis for effective sensorimotor learning ability;

❯ determine the degree of use of fitness abilities;

❯ promote the possibility of learning and relearning, even at an older age;

❯ facilitate the acquisition of sports-technical skills from other sports; and

❯ are the most valuable active injury prophylaxis.

Coordination abilities enable the player to confidently master the predictable and unpredictable in soccer (Weineck, Memmert, and Uhing, 2012, p. 17). Coordination abilities mesh particularly with physical performance factors, analyzing abilities, and already acquired *movement skills, techniques (wealth of movements),* and *movement experiences* with the implementation of the movement. They, thereby, represent a kind of *vehicle* for the *progressive optimization* of the depicted components of a soccer player's performance within a long-term training structure (i.e., base, foundations, basic, advanced, and high-performance training) to be able to utilize, for instance, the following effectively and without injury during playing action:

❯ Reacting and acting quickly

❯ Reading and seeing the game

❯ Acting early to stop a dangerous situation

❯ Being able to fall or roll and get up quickly

❯ Beingthe boss in the air and maintaining control

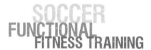

That means

◉ having take off power, balance, and orientation ability and

◉ being able to respond quickly, nimbly, and precisely in all situations.

The power component coordination (and agility) is extremely important to the desired training and playing philosophy. It acts as a kind of link between the main sports motor demands of speed, strength, and endurance and the technical and tactical abilities and skills on and off the ball. Precise and quick control of individual movements while using as much range of motion of the movement apparatus as possible may be viewed as the prerequisite for implementation of the own game concept.

As Weineck, Memmert, and Uhing (2012), in particular, were able to show theoretically and practically in their latest impressive publication on optimal coordination training in soccer based on sports-scientific principles, coordination training is based on the variation principle. It requires that the coach and instructor do the following during the practice and training process:

◉ Offer situations with complex movements.

◉ Be able to feel the sense of movement and its qualitative enhancement and completion from the player's perspective.

◉ Pick up on the player's special needs (e.g., bodyawareness, generating own ideas, movement perception, versatility vs. specialization).

The coach's and instructor's behavioral role is guided by the complexity of the subject: versatile, enthusiastic, credible, and determined, always open to developments and issues that frequently go beyond "strictly soccer." From this develops a kind of free thinking, in spite of the purposeful individual and communal training and practice and versatile and variable training of the different performance factors. In the authors' estimation, the *versatility concept* in the training process of youth players, in particular, represents a stimulus for a significant transfer of learning.

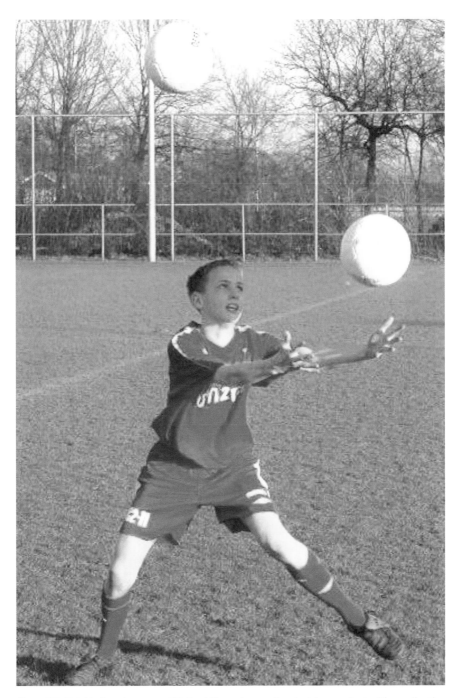

Photo 10: Quickly learning new athletic skills andexpanding training content withcoordination training

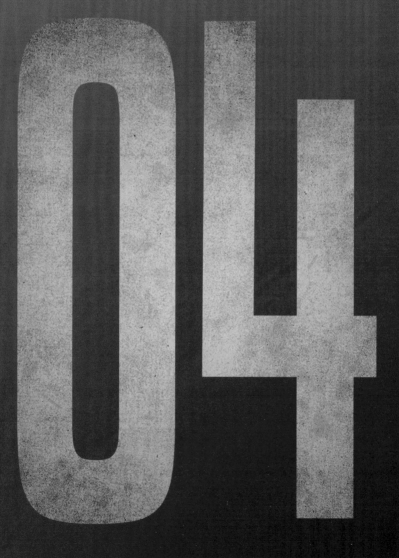

> CHAPTER

04

4 WHICH FACTORS INFLUENCE COORDINATION ABILITIES IN SOCCER?

> *"Coordination-technical abilities under extreme pressure of time, precision, and variability can be seen as the most important components in modern soccer."*

(Weineck, Memmert, and Uhing, 2012, p. 7)

As previously mentioned in chapter 3, coordination abilities are influenced by control and regulating processes during athletic action through the soccer player's analytical abilities, the wealth of movements and experience, and the physical performance factors.

The physical performance factors, in particular, impact the level of coordination ability in soccer. In today's modern competitive play and training, the performance factor of *speed* is of critical importance (see chapter 17). It is determined by subskills that should be optimally developed during a soccer player's long-term training process (see table 1).

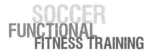
Table 1: Speed subskills of a soccer player (based on Weineck, 2004, p. 378)

A soccer player's speed is determined by:		
	Action speed For example, during 3-on-3 in a small space	Playing together as fast and as effectively as possible (technical, tactical, and coordination requirements)
	Fast action Off the ball, acceleration and deceleration	Executing cyclical and acyclical actions off the ball as fast as possible (sprinting, decelerating, turning, and reversing)
	Reaction speed For example, reaction games with a partner	Quickly reacting to unexpected actions (ball, opponent, teammate)
	Speed of decision-making For example, lots of big and small position games and special game situations	Making an appropriate decision from a multitude of choices in a very short time
	Anticipation speed For example, improved knowledge of the game in terms of performing and contemplating a variety of game situations)	Quick anticipation of play
	Cognitive speed For example, by practicing familiar and unfamiliar game situations	Quickly learning to assess current game situations by means of auditory and visual information

Thus, being able to sprint fast is not just a matter of linking physical performance factors. Rather, the soccer player should possess strength, endurance, and the mindset (in terms of intrinsic motivation) to be able to, for instance, endure such a sprinting program in practice. Furthermore, he needs to have a sense of rhythm and tempo to be able to lengthen or shorten his stride. In a competitive game, this process must sometimes be executed with a low center of gravity since the player must anticipate a shove (shoulder to shoulder) at any moment (see chapter 16.3). Therefore, a soccer player should be able to execute a sprinting duelwith relaxed as well as flexedmuscles. At the same time this puts the player's ability to link motor skills to the test. This reconfirms the high degree of complexity in soccer.

"Defensively I have a certain quality with my head, but offensively I have to hit the goal. But that's not so easy. Sometimes I ask myself how the boys are even able to aim when it is so tight in the opposing penalty box..."

(Nuri Sahin, Borussia Dortmund and player on the Turkish national team, in kicker, March 9, 2015, 22, p. 19)

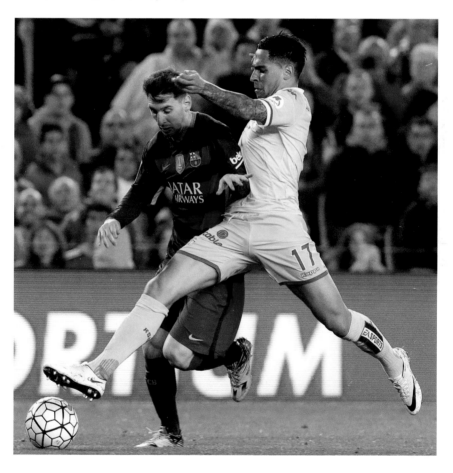

> CHAPTER
05

5 TALENT SUPPORT AS MISSION AND GOAL OF YOUTH DEVELOPMENT IN SOCCER

> *"Based on prevailing opinion, coordination abilities form the basis for motor learning ability, athletic aptitude, or sports-related talent."*

(Roth, 2005, p. 327)

The comments in chapters 2, 3, and 4 emphasize that a versatile training of coordination abilities and factors that influence coordination abilities is of critical importance to individual and optimal performance development in soccer. In the authors' estimation, talent support should follow the principles of goaldirectedness, systematics, continuity, immersion, and progression.[7] According to the current state of sports-science research, the preferred instruction method for the optimization of coordination abilities is through "ball schools," meaning a playful approach combined with a differentiated learning method (Schöllhornet al., 2006; Roth and Kröger, 2011; König, Memmert, and Moosmann, 2012; Weineck, Memmert, and Uhing, 2012; Roth et al., 2013; Roth et al., 2014a; Roth andHegar, 2014b; Schöllhorn, Hegen, and Eckhoff, 2014). Taking into account *educational perspectives* and *methodological suggestions*, this can be summarized for *basic soccer instructionas* done in table 2.

---

7   *See Höhner, 2012, p. 270-271.*

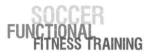

Table 2: Basic soccer instruction in terms of learning by playing a variety of games with a ball[8]

During **basic instruction**, youth soccer players should possess technical, coordinated, and tactical skills and building blocks from a variety of sports games. Youth players should have the opportunity for communal, active, and successful participation in different games. For this reason,the nurturing of *playing intelligence* and *creativity* are at the heart of soccer training.
Playful implicit learning lends itself well.

Training tasks: The goal of the following three approaches is the differentiated and isolated instruction of fundamental, basic tactical, coordinated, and sensorimotor content.

Instruction of offensive and defensive tactical modules from a variety of sports games[9]	*Objective:* To hit the target and to take the ball to the target (e.g., island game, numbers ball) *Partner aspect:* Creating advantages and promoting team play (e.g., mat ball, wall ball) *Opponent aspect:* Recognizing gaps and evading opponent interference (e.g., hand–foot ball game) *Environmental aspect:* Signaling being open and orienting (e.g., contact ball and zone soccer) The *defensive modules* result from reversing the offensive point of view (e.g., preventing hitting the target or closing a gap)
Improving overall ball coordination	*Motor skills* should hereby be learned quickly and precisely, be controlled purposefully and precisely, and be modified versatilely and appropriate situationally. Practicing *informational motor requirement modules* (content) should follow the basic formula: Basic ball skills plus variety plus pressure conditions.
Improving basic ball skills	Establishing *general skill modules* should be at the center of training: controlling angles and direction of play, controlling exertion, determining the point of contact on the ball, determining running lanes and tempo to the ball, getting open, (anticipating passing), playing direction and distance, and anticipating defensive position.

Methods: *Independently finding* anappropriate solution and the ability to generate many solutions. Working on communication rules within the context of social interactions (e.g., listening and not interrupting, learning organizational forms [line-ups], learning to fix and recognize signals, setting up and dismantling equipment together).

---

8 *In 2006, te Poel was able to integrate the underlying concept of basic soccer instruction for sports games into the entire sports curriculum for the state of Hesse, Germany and codify the same together with the commission.*

9 *The extremely important transition play in modern soccer (from defense to offense) is kept in mind here, but not explicitly implemented.*

At present, the many publications by Neumaier and Mechling (1999), Raab (2000), Schöllhorn et al. (2006), Roth and Kröger (2011), and Weineck, Memmert, and Uhing (2012) provide theorized models, drills, and forms of training to optimize coordination with the ball (undirected, across different sports games, and sport game specific).

In the following chapters, the authors will, therefore, focus primarily on the *physical performance factors*, including *coordination training*, in youth soccer instruction.

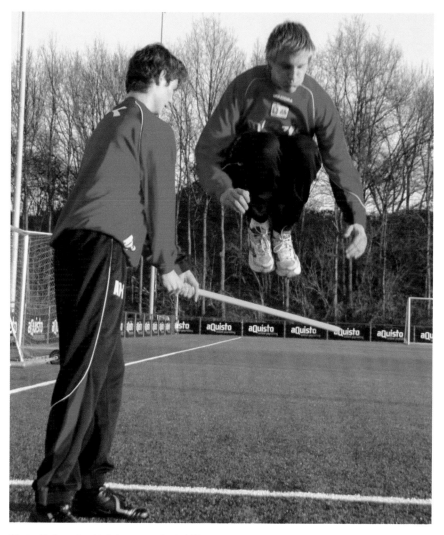

Photo 11: Jumping high is an acquired skill!

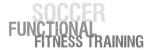

In performance-oriented soccer, the *physical performance factors* are increasingly integrated into soccer training in a performance-enhancing, preventative, and rehabilitative manner, most often by means of an athletic or fitness trainer orthrough additional training and practice units. To the authors' knowledge, a compendium of youth soccer does not exist at this time. We intend to close that gap with this book. Executing techniques and tactics economically and effectively with playful ease to all of our delight and appreciation requires a substantial and broad foundation (see chapter 2, fig. 3).

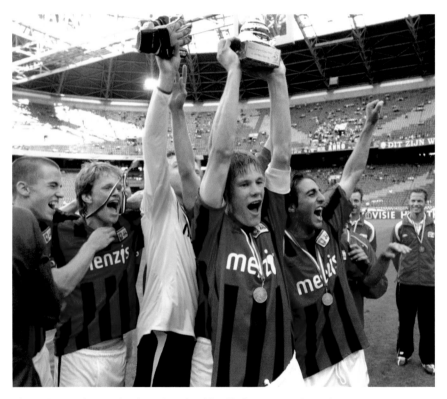

Photo 12: Snapshot: Junior champions, but it's still along way to the top!

This foundation builds on early learning experiences from a variety of movement requirements. In the authors' opinion as well as that of present pertinent literature, insufficient coordination abilities do not result from inadequate abilities, but rather from a lack of encouragement at a young age. When schools and clubs are no longer able to provide the physical performance requirements for various reasons, then the responsible and goal-oriented development with a view to the future in terms of talent search and support and pro soccer instruction, in particular, can become a gamble, including chancefinds from among a quarter billion soccer-playing people worldwide. Reason enough to provide the interested reader this book, based on many years of experience and theoretical principles, for critical consideration.

CHAPTER

06

6 YOUTH TRAINING – VERSATILE, DEVELOPMENTAL, AND VARIED

"An optimal attention span, the phenomenon of laterality, of legpreference, directionality, execution sequence with weak and strong extremities, contralateral transfer, and versatility, are of critical importance to improving coordinated technical abilities in soccer."

(Weineck, Memmert, and Uhing, 2012, p. 73)

When looking at a soccer player's individual development trajectory, one can see that the timing for optimal trainability of fitness-related abilities (i.e., physical performance factors) does not coincide with that of coordination abilities. Due to the quick development of neuromuscular and sensorimotor control and regulation,it is never too soon to begin the trainingof coordination abilities in soccer. It should already be addressed during preschool age by initiating and acquiring movement skills. In the authors' estimation, this considerably increases learning effectiveness and is conducive to a sufficiently developed foundation (see chapter 2, fig. 3; Roth, Hegar, 2014b). Furthermore, Weineck, Memmert, and Uhing (2012, p. 41) point out that "learning perfect motion sequences is already possible during childhood."

When choosing from our drills and forms of play, putting together teams and choosing talents, coaches, and instructors should, as a matter of principle, take into account the following parameters:

- Biological age[10]
- Relative training age
- Gender
- Performance level (test and ball control drills)
- Motivation
- Interest
- Below average andabove average tests and ball control drills

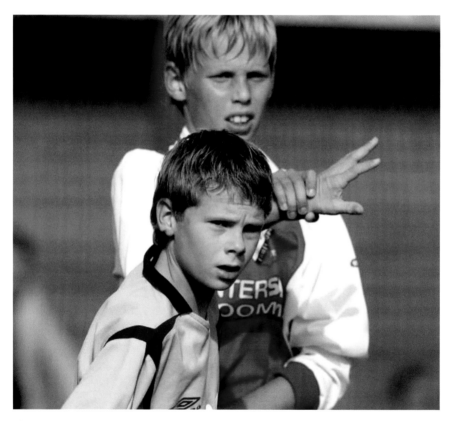

Photo 13: Be aware of biological acceleration. Small players are no less gifted!

10   *At this point we refer to the empirical research by Lames et al. (2008) on "relative age effect" (RAE). Particularly with respect to talent search and selection in soccer, in the future, more consideration should be given to the fact that the minimal developmental edge that relatively older players have within an age group can be amplified by biological acceleration. Moreover, accompanying athletic successes act as a kind of mental motivation booster. Additional support measures, in part, facilitate this process. However, if coaches and instructors pursue the objective that youth training consists of achieving individual top performance during the top-performance age, as do the authors of this book, they must closely analyze the relative age effect, because the assumption is that talent in sports does not depend on a birth date.*

The following criteria should be taken into account with respect to load and stress characteristics:

- ◈ *Stimulus intensity:* How fast am I running?
- ◈ *Stimulus duration:* How long am I playing?
- ◈ *Stimulus volume:* How many miles am I running?
- ◈ *Stimulus density:* What is the ratio of running distance and number of runs to the length of the breaks?
- ◈ *Training methods:* Intensive or extensive interval training, duration method, repeated runs
- ◈ *Training surface:* Grass, synthetic surface, cinders, gym floor, forest soil
- ◈ *Running school:* Uphill, stairs of varying length and height, varying distances
- ◈ Required *training aids?*

The training methodology helps coaches and instructors enormously to convert the individual, group, and team-specific objectives into practical training. In doing so, the variables age and predisposition play an important role.

Until age six, children move *spontaneously, unbridled,* and *informally.* In this phase, objectives and planning and sports game directionality in *sports game communication* are largely unknown to them. Starting at age six, playing is, therefore, a child's most important form of communication and of critical importance and vital to the subsequent development of optimal playing and sports performance—all the way to old age. Sports instruction should, therefore, be geared to the entirety (and game idea) in connection with the respective rules and tasks of the game.

Forms of play on small playing fields (with short passing distances and lots of touches), relays, and fitness parcours with and without competitive aspects make up the content of this training phase. Since children's groups mostly consist of heterogenic and coeducational learning groups, time is limited, and the game means something different to boys than girls. Working with children represents a major technical and educational challenge for coaches and instructors: During this stage of development the individual child should have the opportunity to actively and creatively participate in the game and achieve at least a balanced success–failure record. This training phase is extremely important because here various thinking strategies can be trained efficiently (Roth, Roth, and Hegar, 2014).

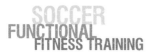

For this reason, the joy of playing should be most important. In the authors' opinion, winning (and thus competing) hardly matters before age 10, but developmental rivalry does. Playing and being playful are basic activities on a lower level (Roth, Roth, and Hegar, 2014).

Components such as time pressure, opponent, and complexity that correspond to the competitive character of the target and goal-oriented soccer game are addedonly with the children's increasing age and development level.

The coach and instructor also play a key role during these stages of development by

❯ making the learning progress visible and tangible for the youth players,even if it is minor;

❯ teaching youth to communicate, accept, and support each other; and

❯ showing that competitive games are not always a race against time (see photos 14 and 15).

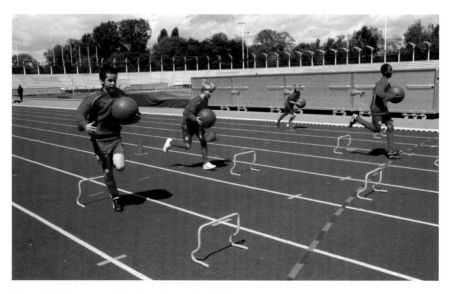

Photo 14: Relay races with obstacles—variety is key

Sequences that emphasize *skill* and *agility* should also be a part of versatile youth training, whereby chance should be an important factor during practice as well the mantra,the "best" one doesn't always win.

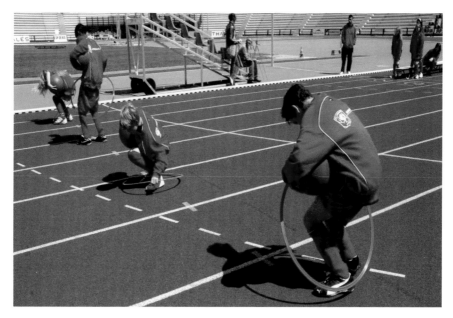

Photo 15: Relays with additional tasks—being able to laugh at oneself!

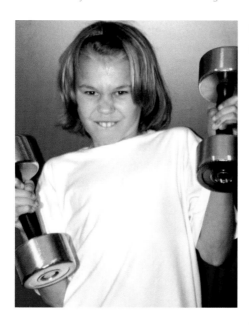

Photo 16: Caution! A child is not a miniature adult.

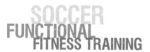

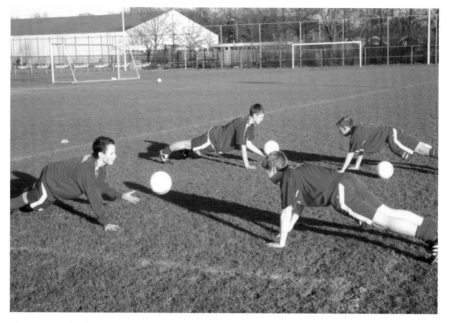

Photo 17: A playful approach is important in youth athletic training: Try throwing the ball from a plank position and catching it with one hand.

It must be said that the choice of content and the methodological approach in training is often influenced by the objectives of the club, the soccer school, the entity, and the curriculum. Objectives should be verbalized consistently and clearly and should be transparent and workable for all participants in the training process. Since, for instance, youth competitive sports centers of the German Bundesliga teams consider achieving individual top performance during top performance age to be at the center of the long-term training process, the individual development level of children and youth players is always the starting point for the didactic, methodological, and educational decisions that coaches and instructors make.

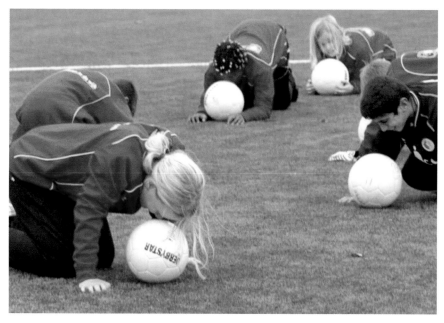

Photo 18: The coach or instructor provides the developmentally appropriate practice material, in which, next to practicing, the joy of "doing" should play a role.

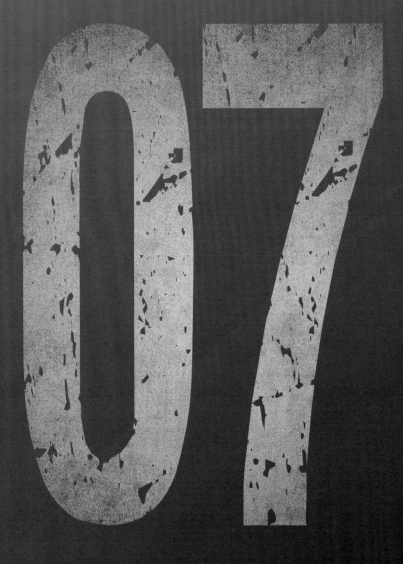

CHAPTER

07

7 DO SOCCER FITNESS AND SOCCER PLAYING HAVE TO BE SEPARATE?

"Soccer fitness before running fitness, and you play the way you train!"

(I.A. to G. Hiddink)

There is empirical evidence that many youth soccer players who flock to clubs or schools increasingly exhibit deficiencies in the main physical fitness components (see Naul et al., 2003, on Finnish and German students).

The most recent study by Greier and Riechelmann (2012) on ball game injuries in Austrian school sports showed that ball sport injuries were more prevalent during physical education. Next to small ball games and basketball, soccer has the most injuries (predominantly distortions). The majority of injuries sustained in school sports ball games tend to be to the upper extremities (p. 168). Greier and Riechelmann assume that coordination weaknesses as well as overuse and lack of basic technical skills are the possible causes.

Furthermore, when following the latest empirical results by Schmitt (2013, p. 18-27), a fundamentally higher injury risk can be ascertained in the contact game sport of soccer:

Approximately a third of all injuries occur without physical contact with an opponent. In more than two-thirds of cases injuries and overuse damages involve the lower extremities. These are primarily upper thigh muscle injuries, followed by knee and ankle injuries. Overuse injuries are frequently seen in the inguinal region. Here we must differentiate between intra- and extra-articular causes. Coxarthrosis is frequently seen in former soccer players as a long-term effect of intensive loading with formation of a femoroacetabular impingement.

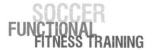

There is still debate in the scientific community as to the extent to which preventative hip surgery can be preformed. Depending on the involvement of internal structures of the knee, direct injuries to the knee have a critical impact on the occurrence of secondary damage. Preventative measures appear to reduce the frequency of injuries (p. 18).

When broadening the test subjects to professional men's soccer and attempting to link the higher number of games with possible effects on performance and playing availability, the results from the latest UEFA injury study can be summarized as follows:

The average injury frequency rate in elite soccer is 3 to 5 injuries per 1000 hours of training, and 25 per 1000 hours of play. On average a team with 25 players can expect 50 injuries per season. The injury rate did not go up during this 11-year period. It varies in European countries with an increased risk of ACLinjuries (anterior cruciate ligament), but an overall lower injury risk in countries with a Mediterranean climate. The most common individual injury is to the ischiocrural musculature. Radiological examinations via MRI or ultrasonography are accompanied by periods of rest. From a radiological perspective, 70% of all ischiocrural muscle injuries dated in pro soccer rate 0 or 1. This means there are no fiber tears at the time of imaging, but still the cause of most absences. Nearly all male top soccer players with ACLinjuries return to full-time soccer, but only after 6-7 months. Stress fractures are not common among soccer players, but are slow to heal. Injury risk on artificial turf is similarly high as playing on grass. A higher number of games results in negative effects on performance and playing availability in athletes (Ekstrand, 2013, p. 5).

Many sports doctors recommend eccentric strength training, integrated coordination training (with emphasis on proprioceptive training), and learning and improving basic ball techniques as *preventative and therapeutic measures* (Mandelbaum et al., 2005; McKeon et al., 2008; Greier and Riechelmann, 2012).

Kleinöder (2009) and Behringer, vom Heede, and Mester (2009) point out that strength training in youth competitive sports (and especially in game sports) should increasingly follow current scientific training concepts (from childhood to high-performance age). These go far beyond the usual stabilization training and provide specific and early preparation of the active and passive locomotor system for intensive loading during puberty and adulthood on an empirical basis.[11]

Souid (2011) was able to prove within the scope of a dissertation on preventative measures in elite soccer that the knee joint's susceptibility to injury is related particularly to the strength of the lower extremities. He, therefore,argues strongly for developmentally appropriate athletic training in the area of strength until age 18.

To this effect we can show the following periodization based on the changes to load characteristics (with an associated high spread in the following data):

Periodisierung des Krafttrainings				
Training cycle	General preparation	Special preparation	Pre-competition phase	Competition phase
Training - goal	Hypertrophic loading tolerance	Maximum strength power	Maximum strength power	Maximum value of perfomance retention
Intensity	Low⟶			⟶ High
Volume	High ⟶ Low			⟶
Repetitions	6-20	4-6	2-4	1-3
Sets	3-6	3-6	2-4	2-4
Training units/day	1-3	1-3	1-2	1
Days/week	3-6	3-4	2-4	1-3
L-U-R*	3 zu 1/ 2 zu 1	3 zu 1/ 2 zu 1	3 zu 1/ 2 zu 1	–

*L-U-R =Load–Unload–Rhythm

---

11 *The interested reader can find additional information on the homepage of the Deutsches Forschungszentrum für Leistungssport Köln – momentum (www.dshs-koeln.de/momentum).*

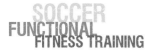

Thus, based on this data, demanding modern youth training that offers a greater presence of versatile and varied training in clubs and schools inthe future, particularly with respect to the physical performance factors, is justified. The fact that the internationally renowned *AJAXtraining school for the training of youth players in top-performance competitive sports* has had judo[12] on their training schedule for some time now, and recently added a spacious *athletic skills outdoor training facility*[13] makes it clear that an ambitious soccer training (and school sports training) should include versatile athletic soccer fitness.

When also looking at the development (and increase) of running intensities and volumes in pro soccer (Siegle et al., 2012) and the fitness levels of youth players (Meyer et al., 2005), the preeminent importance of soccer fitness that permanently accompanies athletes in youth soccer training[14] (and especially beyond that) becomes plausible:

> *It is apparent that the changes in parameters that are relevant to physical performance in adolescent soccer players between the ages of 14 and 18 are primarily due to physical growth. For this reason specific fitness stimuli, particularly in the areas of speed and strength, are needed no later than age 16, to ensure continued progression of the physical foundation of soccer-specific skills* **(Meyer et al., 2005, p. 20).**

Furthermore, Hottenrott and Neumann (2010, p. 13-19) emphasize the importance of loading and unloading through increasing training loads in modern high-performance sports and in the following table 4, tellingly highlight how extensive muscle and performance loss can be with interruption to training.

There is a decrease in muscle strength and even changes in organs, particularly during the off-season,and interruptions in training due to injury, which can also be seen in youth competitive soccer. In pro soccer they should be delayed through corrective strength exercises and suitable cross-training (a different sport) and, thus, help to ensure the athlete's continued overall capacity.

---

12 *Feldbusch, te Poel, and Herborn, 2015.*

13 *Search YouTube for "Athletic Skills Tour."*

14 *A feasible example for the improvement of speed abilities as part of training in a youth training facility was offered by youth trainer Kai Braun in a topical contribution in **fussball training** (2014).*

Table 4: De-adaptation or immobilization due to interruptions in training (based Hottenrott and Neumann, 2010, p. 18)

Days without training	Systems, abilities, and performance	Changes
3-5 days (IT)	Increased resting heart rate (HR) andduring submaximal loading	+3 to +10 BPM
5 days (TU)	Decreased glycogen synthesis activity	−42%
5 days (SL)	Decreased slow-twitch muscle area	−6 to −8%
10 days (TU)	Decreased activity of muscle oxidative enzymes	−23 to −45%
11 days (SL)	Decreased slow-twitch muscle area	−16 to −45%
12 days (BR)	Decreased VO2max. Decreased stroke volume	−7% −11%
14 days (BR)	Decreased size of slow-twitch fibers	−12 to −15%
14 days (TU)	Increased submaximal heart rate	+10 BPM
14 days (TU)	Electrical activity in muscles	−3 to −13%
17 days (BR)	Decreased thin muscle filament (actin) Thick filaments (myosin) unchanged Loss of maximal strength (MS)	−16 to −23% −13%
17 days (SL)	Atrophy of slow-twitch and fast-twitch fibers Diminished strength Decreased absolute strength	−6%
21 days (TU)	Loss of muscle mass, submaximal and maximal stroke volume as well as VO2max.	−1 to −5% −25% −7 to −27%
28 days (TU)	Decreased strength endurance	−7 to −14%
Impact of bed rest (BR), zero gravity (ZG), and (injury-induced) interruption of training (IT) on performance and functional systems.		

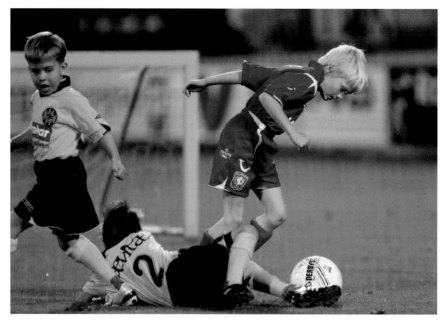

Photo 19: Falling down, getting up, and keeping balance all are components of children's mini-games. These abilities and skills are part of the game of soccer and must be learned and mastered (see chapter 16.3).

CHAPTER 08

8 FROM SOFT SKILLS TO TRAINING DIFFERENT AGE GROUPS

> *"As a coach one naturally hopes to contribute to their [youth competitive player] advancement. In any case, based on personal experience, I can say that it is a lot of fun to make progress together."*

(H. Geschwindner, personal trainer, advisor, and mentor of superstar Dirk Nowitzki, from an interview with Eva Pfaff, 2013, p. 50)

It is important to know that accelerated and delayed players must be carefully evaluated with respect to their level of training and future development,using not only the screening and scouting of youth players, but also their **performance** which often also provides conclusions about training content and playing positions. Whether ectomorph and leptosome, or mesomorph and athlete, or endomorph and pyknic type, when regarded very carefully, this typecasting can provide additional information for the assessment of physical performance factors and coordination abilities.

This also applies to the physiological and psychological development characteristics that facilitate a differentiated performance evaluation and development from early (ages 6-10) and late (ages 10-13) childhood, through puberty (ages 12-15) and adolescence (ages 15-18), all the way to adulthood (Memmert, Weineck, and Uhing, 2012, p. 41-44).

Moreover, prior to their screening and planning,coaches and instructors should be careful to take into account the basic needs of youth players. Often it is the *soft skills* that can negatively impact the development of physical performance factors and coordination abilities in spite of optimal institutional and personnel conditions and training guidelines.

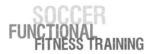

The job of a coach orinstructor is not to support the playerpermanently. Rather, he should make sure that the player doesn't need support.

Being aware of the fundamental needs of young soccer players is also conducive to the social responsibility to foster independence and self-fulfillment as coaches and instructors and to better classify training within the different age groups. Based on the Maslow pyramid (Miller, Vandome, and Mc Brewster, 2010), this aspect can be outlined as follows (see fig. 4):

**Indepen-
dence
and self-
reliance**

**Self-development and
self-fulfillment**
within a demanding and facili-
tative training climate

Appreciation and acknowledgment
lends self-confidence

Protection and security
as a guarantee for "free" and joyful playing and
training

Social interaction
at the soccer club and within the team creates a sense of belon-
ging, secures personal status, and facilitates empathy

Participation in family and social life
acquiring adequate basic nutrition and clothing, developmentally-approp-
riate housing conditions and hygiene (rest, medical care), nicotine-, drug-, and
alcohol-free environment; living in a family or family-like structure (e.g., boarding
school); being able to play sports and manage time and exposure to new media and a
future-oriented education

Fig. 4: Soft skills—the ambitious training kit

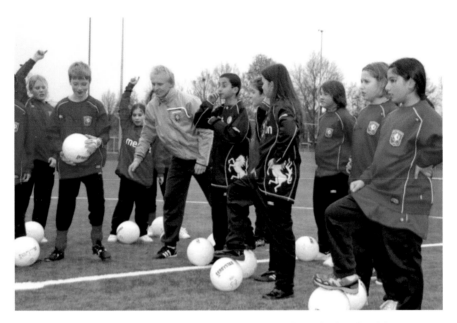

Photo 20: A safe and trusting training atmosphere is the starting point for all training.

Building on this, cognitive[15] and socio-affective factors[16] should also be analyzed prior to creating a master plan for training physical performance factors and coordination abilities in youth players.

Meeting youth players in training at their actual level should not just be an empty phrase.

---

15 *The authors hereby link soccer knowledge and academic performance.*

16 *Lifestyle and well-being in a general sense.*

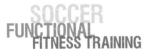
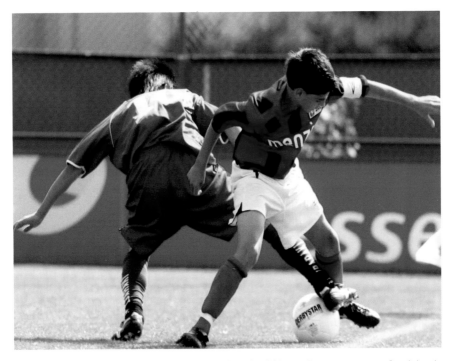

Photo 21: Fair battle for the ball—stability training should be an important part—of training in every age group.

An exemplary rough draft of the structure of training content in the form of a *youth player master plan* based on *"tua res agitur"* (it concerns you), regarding actual prerequisites, the intended playing and training philosophy, and a code of conduct can subsequently be created for training physical performance factors and coordination abilities. Hereafter the authors will orient themselves by the known developmental characteristics (Martin et al., 1999, p. 25-64) and the DFB's (German Football Association) and the KNVB's (Royal Dutch Football Association) valid age group classifications. The *basic principle of timely and increasing specialization* will also be taken into consideration, whereby the ontogenetic as well as the training-related dependency of training effects must be understood. At this point, we will forgo the popular proportioning and block structure (with block-specific goals) of general and specific training content[17] on the timeline of the long-term performance development in favor of an outline of general guidelines for specified abilities and

---

17 *General training results from individual prerequisites. Specific training results from the systematic development of sport-specific performance requirements.*

practice-oriented goals and examples (summaries) within the associations' valid age groups. But at this point it must be stated as a matter of principle that (during the periods of *advanced* and *high-performance training*)

◉ during childhood (early and late), a high demand on information-receiving and processing systems, and

◉ an accelerated speed development until the start of puberty

can be ascertained.

The stage of training until the onset of puberty can be referred to as the *phase of versatile athletic preparation.*

A marked increase in the demand on the body's energy-related processes and an increase in the specific training content portion can be noted during *advanced training* and *high-performance training.*

Furthermore, *constitutional characteristics,* the nature of the loading capacity (organic, mechanical, mental), and interplay between performance requirements [18]relevant for transferability must always be kept in mind.

---

18 *The extent to which coordination abilities, speed, strength, and endurance affect each other and are linked depends on the **degree of utilization of neuromuscularperformance requirements** (i.e., coordination abilities heavily draw on cognitive performance requirements; in contrast endurance abilities are more likely to utilize energy-related organic performance requirements).*

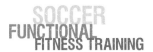

Table 5: General guidelines for endurance, strength, speed, and coordination abilities (and agility) for U7 players (ages 5-8)[19]

Developmental characteristics	Endurance	Strength[20]
Physical • Improved coordination abilities increase utilization of strength. • Harmonic movements. • Feel for the ball is barely perceptible and developed. • Enormous urge to move. • Balance is smooth. **Cognitive** • Short concentration phases. • Moderate competitiveness. • Game is an adventure. • Discovery of own potential (imagination). **Socio-affective** • Little cooperation.	Continuous exertion at low intensity is well suited. Use a variety of forms of play and drills. Keep training volume low.	Strength increases with versatile forms of play and drills.

SUMMARY

STRENGTH

Objective: Specific muscle strength does not exist yet. Better functional muscle strength will be initiated by improved general coordination.

Drills: Lots of forms of play with small obstacles. No systematic jumping exercises.

ENDURANCE

Objective: Endurance training at low intensity and in playful form is possible.

---

19 *The KNVB identifies its youth players as pupils, including the mini-pupils (bambini) who play exclusively 4-on-4 games.*

20 *Regarding the use of the terms **strength** and **athletic training**, the authors refer to the introduction (p. 16-17).*

Speed	Coordination
Speed increases with imaginative play and selection of drills.	Agility is highly developed. Motor learning gains are clearly going up. Simple and new motor skills are quickly absorbed and learned. Differentiation inhibition is still insufficient. Lack of movement accuracy and quality of spatial–temporal structural features.

Forms of play: Continuous exertion of 1 minute (e.g., 4 x 1 minute) followed by short breaks

SPEED

Objective: Starting at ages 5 and 6, increased speed of movement coincides with improved coordination. Reaction speed can be positively developed.

Forms of play: Different forms of play and reaction games with emphasis on sensorimotor skills: tactile, visual, acoustic.

COORDINATION AND AGILITY

Objective: Agility can easily be developed, and motor learning gains increase between ages 5 and 6. Simple abilities and skills can be learned easily.

Drills: Lots of rhythmic drills with versatile movement. Development of basic running, jumping, and throwing skills.

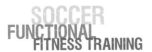

Table 6: General guidelines for endurance, strength, speed, and coordination abilities (and agility) for youth players (U9/U8, ages 8-10)

Developmental characteristics	Endurance	Strength
Physical • Physique is more even. As a result, coordination and functional strength increase. **Cognitive** • Learning is initiated. • Increasing awareness to take on tasks. • Good age for motor learning processes. **Socio-affective** • Increased social and group consciousness. • Still limited concentration phases. Flexibility in use of content and methods is advised.	Endurance ability can be improved using partisan games and low-intensity drills. Approximately 10-minute duration per position game should not be exceeded. Children may themselves choose lower intensities in a game.	Strength increases through many different movement experiences. Power is initiated through easy jumping games like hopscotch and skipping. Preparation for strength exercises is done by increasing number of jumps, for example.

SUMMARY

STRENGTH

Objective: Continued development of functional strength through more movement experiences. Explosive and takeoff power can be partially improved.

Drills: Skipping and small jumps over small obstacles. No strength endurance exercises.

ENDURANCE

Objective: Aerobic endurance capacity increases. Focus is on the sense of tempo and movement technique.

Exercises: Should be of a playful nature. Active breaks are longer than 2 minutes.

Forms of play: 4 x 2 minutes, or 3 x 3 minutes, or 2 x 4 minutes, or series of 3 minutes – 3 minutes – 2 minutes, or 1 minute – 2 minutes – 3 minutes – 2 minute – 1 minute loading duration.

Speed	Coordination
The acceleration process is activated and advanced through speed exercises (reaction games and short sprints in relays).	Coerver techniques and a large selection of forms of play and drills help to improve coordination abilities. The feel for the ball improves and can be facilitated using simple ball-mastery drills. Perfecting reaction ability, the ability to perform high-frequency movements, spatial differentiation ability, coordination under pressure of time, and balance.

SPEED

Objective: Between ages 7 to 9, the basic characteristics of an effective running technique increase, and the range of speed exercises should be expanded. Reaction ability improves at age 9 and movement frequency increases considerably.

Forms of play and drills: Continue forms of play; conscious movement instruction through frequency training with hoops and poles.

COORDINATION AND AGILITY

Objective: Agility continues to increase. Basic motor skills continue to develop by increasing differentiation based on movement forms. Now soccer-specific techniques can be initiated.

Drills: Expansion of technical abilities and skills by means of different movement combinations in different situations.

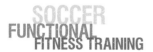

Table 7: General guidelines for endurance, strength, speed, and coordination (and agility) abilities for youth players (U11/U10; ages 10 to 12)

Developmental characteristics	Endurance	Strength
Physical • Often marked differences between early and late developers. • Lots of drive to perform. • Start of puberty. • Limbs grow disproportionatelyat times. **Cognitive** • Emergence of an attitude toward the sport. **Socio-affective** • Formation of ego identity and a sense of group affiliation. • Knows and recognizes others' feelings and adapts to them. • Learns to adapt to environment. Feels dependent and wants to be independent. This can result in recognizable pubertal overreactions.	Improved endurance through extensive interval training of 10-12 minutes (e.g., by means of forms of positional play).Development of feel for tempo and running. Intensive alactic and lactic training should be avoided.	At this age there is a recognizable improvement in the load–strength ratio. Practice with bodyweight. Mobility and strength exercises to even out imbalances are evident. .

Speed	Coordination
Improved speed due to versatile coordination training. *Objective:* Inter- and intramuscular coordination. U11 and U10 players are already able to perform exercises with a high movementfrequency. With the approach of puberty, the frequency response changes, resulting in sometimes major differences. In training, more emphasis is, therefore, placed on differentiation and individualization.	Good learning opportunity for children who are not yet in the (steep) growth phase. Youth players who are in a growing phase have problems learning during unfamiliar coordination exercises. The movements are characterized by abrupt and halting execution. Learning by example, therefore, plays an important role (keyword mirror neurons). Expanding the wealth of movements is, therefore, critical to the development of movement skills.

SUMMARY

STRENGTH

Objective: Improved strength capacity. Explosive power improves parallel to improved speed.

Drills: Skipping and running jumps over and around obstacles. Double-leg jumps. No series. Generate lots of fun in training and forms of play.

ENDURANCE

Objective: Continued increase in aerobic endurance capacity. Systematic training makes cardiovascular adaptations possible. Improved running technique and sense of tempo result in an improved running ability. The following loads are recommended.

Length of breaks: Longer than 2 minutes.

Forms of play: Specify in minutes: 5-4-3-2-1, or 4-3-3-2-2, or 5 x 2 minutes, or 2 x 5 minutes, or 4 x 3 minute, or 3 x 4 minutes loading duration.

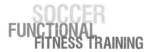

SPEED

Objective: Movements become more dynamic. Various techniques reintegrated into the overall sequence of movements. This can result in an improved movement frequency.

Drills: Further frequency development through conscious and subconscious running instruction and by means of ladders, hoops, and poles.

COORDINATION AND AGILITY

Objective: Good developmental opportunities in the areas of feel for the ball, reaction, balance, and rhythmic ability.

Drills: Intensified learning of basic soccer-specific techniques paired with major demonstration skills (e.g., by means of Coerver Coaching). Offer versatile drills that enhance learning (e.g., using Schöllhorn's differential learning model).

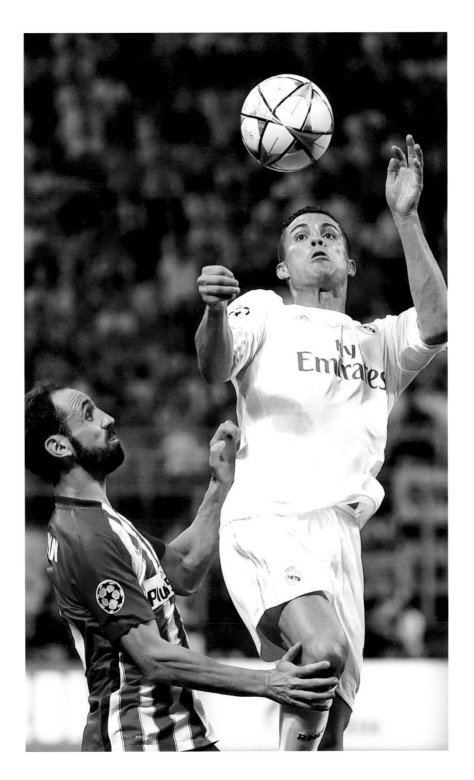

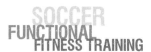

Table 8: General guidelines for endurance, strength, speed, and coordination (and agility) abilities for youth players (U13/U12; ages 12 to 14)

Developmental characteristics	Endurance	Strength
Physical • Development of primary and secondary sexual characteristics begins. • Strength development due to hormonal changes (increased testosterone). • Sudden increase in height and growth. **Cognitive** • Increased questioning and ability to self-reflect. **Socio-affective** • Appearance of negative body image. • Some moodiness. • Striving for independence and responsibility. • Occasional detachment from parents. • Searching for ego-identity. • Group affiliation. • Comparing oneselfto rolemodels.	• Designing versatile training through a good selection of drills and organizational forms: controlled soccer-specific exercises of 12-15 minute durations in cyclical aerobic and alactic form (positional play and partisan games).	• Strength and athletic training using bodyweight and additional light weights is recommended (e.g., medicine balls). Single- and double-leg takeoff strength training on a surface that isn't too hard (e.g., sand: improves support apparatus stability). Vertical and horizontal jumps are acceptable, but without high impact,meaning, no maximal height and distance jumps at high intensity and with frequent repetitions. Lots of attention on development of core strength stability (stomach, back) as well as the arms. Keeping a close eye on growth phases and modifying training as necessary.

Speed	Coordination
No sprint repeats with short breaks. Avoid negative effects on vegetative nervous system. Use running ABCs: emphasis on high movement frequency with and without directional changes (cyclical/acyclical). Stability exercises should be practiced in conjunction with the running ABCs. Frequently change exercise and training equipment (e.g., poles, wide or narrow ladders, hoops, foam blocks). Forms of play and drills with or without a ball with maximally 5- to 20-meter sprints. Be mindful of individual fatigue limits.	Basic ABCs of running and jumping exercises to improve jumping coordination (running fast means jumping fast) and starts and sprints from different positions. From a prone or supine position, long or short sitting position, squat, standing with complete or half turn, after impact or jump are important drills that help improve dexterity combined with sprinting. New movement tasks are learned increasingly faster and better.

SUMMARY

STRENGTH

Objective: Specific differences between the sexes begin to manifest in strength development. Girls possess two-thirds of the strength potential of boys. Beginning at ages 14 to 15, the difference becomes maximal in the strength component.

Drills: Stabilization exercises for the pelvic area and especially stomach and back muscles.

Jumping load: 6-8 jumps left and right; 6-10 running jumps; 6 jumps over small obstacles.

ENDURANCE

Objective: Starting at age 12, differences in the sexes manifest themselves. Aerobic endurance can continue to be developed extremely well.

Length of breaks: More than 2 minutes.

Forms of play: 3 x 5 minutes, or 4 x 4 minutes, or 5 x 3 minutes, or 6 x 2 minutes, or 2 x 6/7 minutes, or (specify in minutes) 6-5-4-3-2-1 or 2-3-4-5-3-2 load duration.

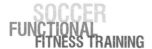

SPEED

Objective: Beginning of optimal speed. Boys are able to purposefully use their strength and thereby improve the *power component speed*.

Drills: Conscious training of techniques. Use of running ABCs.

Speed training: 6-8 x 10-meter sprints from various positions or 6 x 5-meter shuttle run.

COORDINATION AND AGILITY

Objective: First signs of stagnation in technical abilities and skills. Level can continue to go up using specific technical training. Absolute motor learning decreases, but not for certain movement techniques that have already been mastered.

Drills: Many agility exercises with different equipment or with a partner. Repeating and intensifying soccer-specific techniques that have already been mastered. Varying organizational forms. Varying technical training.

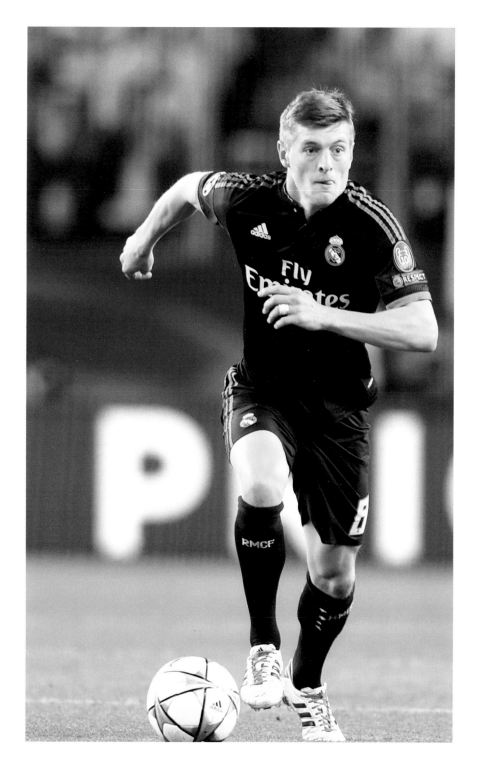

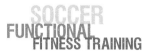

Table 9: General guidelines for endurance, strength, speed, and coordination (and agility) abilities for youth players (U15/U14; ages 14 to 16)

Developmental characteristics	Endurance	Strength
Physical • Development of sexual characteristics due to hormones. • Latedevelopers may suddenly grow. • Strength development increases considerably. **Cognitive** • Continued increase in abstraction and self-reflection abilities. **Socio-affective** • Childhood ends with puberty. • The search for self-identity continues. • Looking to role models and striving for responsibility and independence increases. • Participation in search for solutions. • Steadfastness and sense of reality increase. • Beginning of long-term contacts and friendships. • Search for originality. • Friends are important. • Experimentation increases. • Identifying with things familiar.	• Acyclical aerobic and alactic training within the scope of general soccer-specific forms. The maximum time of approximately 15 minutes for positional games can now be implemented. Lactic anaerobic loads should be kept as low as possible.	• Strength and athletic training can be done using bodyweight, medicine balls, or light freeweights. Additional strength training should be done in cases of muscle and strength deficiencies. General and targeted jumpingABCs.Single-leg or double-leg jumping exercises, whereby emphasis should be placed on gaining space and height. Jumping should be viewed as a means of strengthening familiar soccer-specific thrusting, pulling, hopping, and tackling movements. This should stimulate strength development and anticipative behavior during tackles. In general, stabilizing forms of core exercise should be performed.

SUMMARY

Due to the very different developmental processes of youth players we will forgo explicit suggestions for this age group.

Speed	Coordination
Basic forms of the running ABCs with emphasis on high movement frequency and realistic directional changes, whereby sudden stops, twists, and turns should also be performed. Specific suggestions regarding technique should be made. Use forms of play and drills (between 5-25 minutes with or without ball) that require quick reactions. Caution! Too many repetitions of short sprints lower the speed potential and hamper the development of maximal sprinting speed.	The entire running and jumping repertoire (ABCs) should be usedduring practice and, therefore, takes on an important role. Also included should be exercises with stops and directional changes and combinations thereof in complex game situations: sprinting after jumping, thrusting, falling, and getting up.

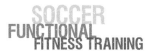
Table 10: General guidelines for endurance, strength, speed, and coordination (and agility) abilities for youth players (U19/U18/U17/U16; ages 16 to 18).

Developmental characteristics	Endurance	Strength
Physical • Physical appearance becomes more adult-like. • Organ systems are well developed. • Physical improvements can be achieved through purposeful and methodically well-planned training. • Peak of motor ability training. **Cognitive** • Abstract thinking is highly developed. • Character building continues. • Increasing self-criticism and need for admiration. • Striving for shared responsibility. **Socio-affective** • Progress in problem-solving process with respect to steadfastness and sense of reality. • Beginning of long-term contacts (friendships). • Increasing self-reliance. • Search for originality. • Friendships are extremely important. • Experimentation decreases. • Identifying with role models.	Prepared and preplanned aerobic training with cyclical and acyclical elements within the scope of soccer-specific exercises. Partisan and positional games of up to approximately 15 minutes are beneficial. Practice of position-specific and individual features.	General and specific strength training with free weights to achieve effective progression with the goal of fast sprinting, stopping, jumping, tackling, and winning. Secondary aspect: Impulses for self-confidence. General and individual strength training with preparation and follow-up.Versatile but targeted strength and athletic training. Different sprinting forms to develop explosive strength by means of static, dynamic, and plyometric exercises. Frequently performing technical, coordination training after strength and athletic training for the purpose ofmomentum transfer.

Speed	Coordination
Multifunctional approach to sprinting with emphasis on frequency, length of passes, and tackles. Increased attention on practicing deceleration movements.Forms of play and drills with strength components and maximal sprints with and without the ball at distances of 5 to 25 meters.Constant focus on and further development ofspeed through special sprint training.	Completion of entire running and jumping ABCs combined with turns, falling, thrusting, and coordination training as complex practice. Adolescence phase makes unrestricted coordination training with higher gains in movement execution, motor control, adaptation and adjustment abilities, and perception possible.

SUMMARY

STRENGTH
STARTING AT AGE 15

Objective: Maximal strength and explosive strength increase in boys. Endurance capacity also increases. This ability should be trained starting now. Basic techniques for specific training (and classic strength training) can now be performed. Strength development in girls levels out.

Drills: Jumping and stabilization exercises of all types.

ENDURANCE
STARTING AT AGE 15

Objective: In 15- to 16-year-old girls, the cardiovascular system is fully developed. In boys, development is not complete until ages 18 to 22. Aerobic endurance capacity can be trained in all its forms. Anaerobic loads can be used starting at age 16.

Forms of play: 3 x 7 minutes, or 3 x 8 minutes, or 3 x 10 minutes, or 10-8-6-4 minutes, or 6 x 4-5 minutes, or 5 x 5-6 minutes load duration.

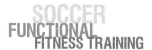

SPEED

STARTING AT AGE 15

Objective: Maximal development of speed and differences between the sexes continue to increase. Strength development levels out in girls and increases in boys. Increased strength as well as improved technique allows the different forms of speed to be further developed through targeted and conscious sprint training.

Drills: Examples: 4 x 10-meter sprints or 4 x 15-meter shuttle runs.

COORDINATION

STARTING AT AGE 15

Objective: In boys, the execution of movement techniques is more dynamic due to the increased strength. Agility increasingly diminishes.

Forms of play and drills: Technique can be improved and further optimized through versatile practice. A variety of choices with different game and movement situations. Put emphasis on agility.

Moreover, depending on the level of training and developmental phase, fitness training should be supplemented with individual training plans: suggestions for relaxation techniques, stabilization and complementary exercises, functional stretching programs, and training aids.

In adults, based on the trained abilities, detail-related improvementsin the area of tactical fitness should take place. The degree of individualization and specificity of a position increase particularly from a coordinated–technical and technical–tactical perspective.

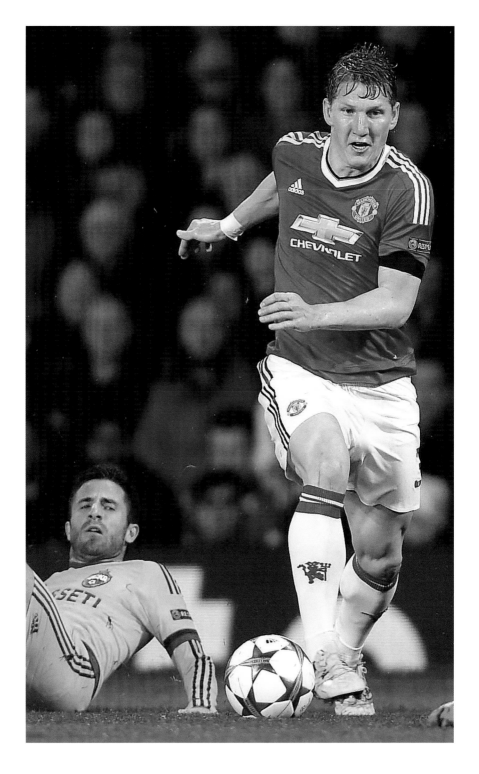

> CHAPTER

09

9 RUNNING, JUMPING, AND THROWING – A SOCCER PLAYER'S BASIC MOTOR ABILITIES

> *"In game sports training—maybe not as extreme as in compositional sports—there is the danger of premature specialization."*

(Steinhöfer, professor of sports science and former prosoccercoach, 2003, p. 9)

In the following chapter we will try to make suggestions to coaches and instructors for the practical organization of ability guidelines (see chapter 8). This will not include, though, an exact allocation to developmental phases and age groups (Weineck, 2004).

9.1 FORMS OF INTRODUCING A TRAINING UNIT

Starting at age 10, a structured and calmly executed warm-up program is beneficial and expedient, especially from the perspective of sports medicine and training and exercise science.

This is not really the case for the youngest players. For this reason,*warm-up games* have become prevalent in soccer. But these can also be used as *cool-down games* at the end of a training unit. Games that include physical contact are very popular with children (and also very soccer appropriate).

In the planning and execution of this training unit, the following didactic guidelines, methodological decisions, and coaching elements proved effective in the field:

- Calmly explain the game and offer examples.
- Focus on one form of introduction.

- Keep organizational forms (e.g., discussion groups, choices) in mind.

- Mark a playing field that has no safety hazards.

- Observe all aspects of safety and support.

- Try to involve all players in the game.

- Keep the chance of winning equal for all participants. This inspires enthusiasm for success.

- Keep in mind your demeanor and tone of your voice. We want to get children excited, not startle or scare them.

- Whenever possible, be physically active as a coach. Avoid sitting down or other positions that might exude distance or even indifference about the chosen form to children and parents.

- As coach, make sure you have a good overview of the game and playing field.

- Address the entire group when making corrections or giving suggestions.

- When necessary, also issue individual instructions.

- Use breaks or rest periods to give tactical advice and ask questions.

- Motivate the children to find their own solutions, stimulations, and improvement suggestions.

- Always ask about the results. Children are sensitive to that.

- Choose games that relate to the children's scope of experience and movement and their fitness-related andcoordinated–technical and tactical qualifications.

- Ensure a precise structure, meaning, start with simple games.

- Whenever possible, choose a game that ties into the last training unit.

- Possibly ramp up the game by involving more children. You can also run several forms simultaneously.

- Provide breaks for the active children (e.g., catchers)—the caught player becomes the catcher.

- Be mindful of issuing points: "When someone touches you, you get a penalty point, but you keep playing!"

- Children should never be ejected from the game!

- Make sure that the game is not too long. Make sure the group always stays on task.

9.2 CATEGORIES OF WARM-UP OR COOL-DOWN GAMES

The authors divide warm-up or cool-down games into three categories. The criteria for classification are based on the objectives of the different forms:

First category: Specific running lane
Second category: Forms of teamwork
Third category: Skillfully negotiated obstacles

9.2.1 SPECIFYING THE RUNNING LANE – CATCHING GAMES

The original form in this category is the game of catch during school recess. This game has many variations and group-specific, problem-solving approaches. The following forms work well on the soccer field or in the gym.

EXERCISE 1: CATCH ME!

One or two catchers are positioned on the centerline of a marked field (9 x 8 m). The catching game begins with a signal from a child or the coach or instructor. Players can start from both sides of the field. Beware of possible collisions. Anyone who is caught (i.e., touched) can return "catch." See who can achieve the most touches during a specified amount of time. The focus of this form is spatial orientation.

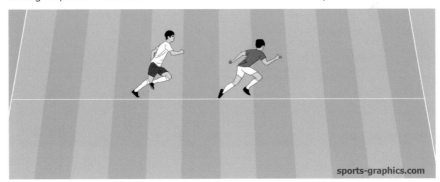

Fig. 5: Two players play catch on the centerline.

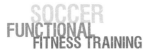

EXERCISE 2: TEAMWORK

Create a game of catch with one pair of players and one hunted player in the center. Work with your partner. When the hunted player is touched, the pairs change. See which player receives the fewest touches. Specify a time period.

EXERCISE 3: VARIATIONS OF CATCHING GAMES

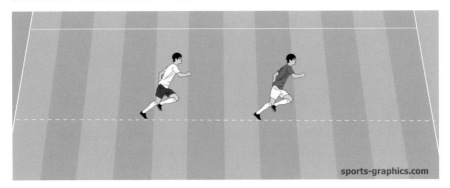

Fig. 6: Game of catch on the lines of a volleyball court.

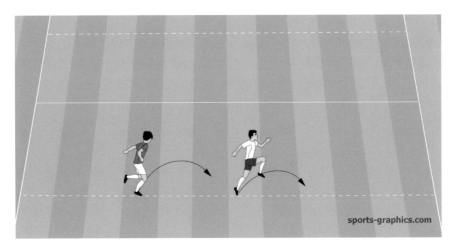

Fig. 7: Single-leg game of catch between the centerlines of a volleyball court.

EXERCISE 4: THE GREAT WALL OF CHINA

Several players attempt to get from one side of a volleyball court (see fig. 7) to the other. One catcher is positioned on the centerline and tries to touch the players. If he succeeds, the player he touches forms a sort of wall with the catcher, and now both of them try to stop and touch the other players. Every player who is touched must become a part of the wall. The players who try to change sides can also "flee" through the wall (but without being touched). Determine number of players and apply the following rules:

1. Catching for a specified period of time or until all have been caught.
2. Change sides after a specified period of time (count number of changes).

EXERCISE 5: DEAL!

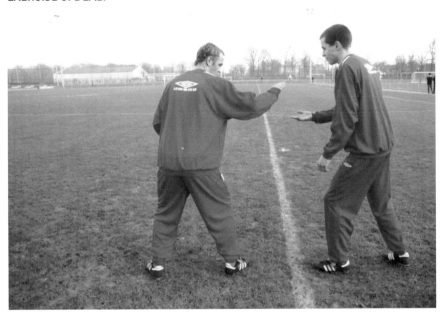

Photo 22: Deal! Who reacts quickest?

Two players face each other, separated by a line. The right player extends his hand. The left player slaps the open palm and sprints toward a marked line behind his back. Immediately after the hand slap, the second player tries to touch the back of the bolting player. The sprinting duel ends when one player reaches the marked line or is touched on the back. Change tasks. Possible scoring methods:

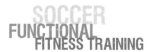

a) Each touch is worth a bonus point. See who is the first to score three bonus points.

b) Each sprint across the line is worth a bonus point. See who is the first to score three bonus points.

c) Each touch is awarded a penalty point and each won sprint duel is awarded a bonus point. See who is the first to score three bonus points.

Specify sprinting distances according to training and teaching goals.

VARIATION

❯ Start: Play in a seated or kneelingposition.

EXERCISE 6: MESSI VS. LAHM

Likeexercise 5, several pairs can participate here. The players in one group are the Messies, and the others are the Lahms. When the coach or instructor calls out Messi, all of the Messies sprint toward the line marked behind them. The Lahms must now touch the Messies during the sprint before the Messies cross the line. The sprint can also start from a

❯ squat,
❯ long seat—facing each other,
❯ long seat—back to back,
❯ cross-legged position,
❯ backward-facingplank,
❯ forward-facing plank,
❯ prone position, or
❯ supine position.

Scoring is the same as exercise 5. Specify sprint distances according to the training and teaching goal.

EXERCISE 7: SPEED CATCHER

One catcher must touch as many players as possible within a specified time period and within a marked playing field. Players who have been touched continue to play.

See how many players you can touch. Create a ranking list.

VARIATIONS:

a) Players can only be touched in a certain order, such as 4-3-2-1-0.

b) The touch is replaced by a tug on the jersey or bib, like in flag football.

EXERCISE 8: THE CHANGER

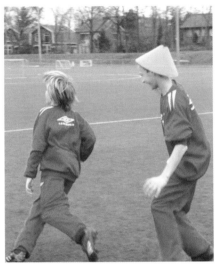

Photo 23: The catcher is easily recognizable.

Field size is approximately 15 x 15 meters, depending on the number of players.

Compare to exercise 7: The player who has been touched becomes the new catcher. The catcher wears a clearly visible hat or marking hood or carries a wooden or plastic staff or a ball. The equipment is constantly passed off and received. Tasks change as soon as a player leaves the field. Playing time, field size, and number of teammates and catchers are determined based on the training and teaching goal.

See how often you are the catcher.

EXERCISE 9: THE HOOP

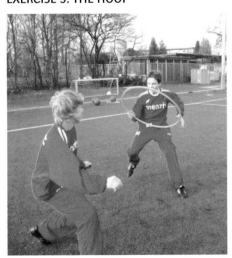

Photo 24: It's all about dexterity and anticipation.

Compare to exercise 8: On a playing field that is 15x 15 meters, the catcher tries to place a hoop over another player's head with one or both hands. If he succeeds, they switch tasks.

See which player scores the fewest goals.

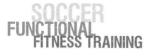

EXERCISE 10: BATTLEFIELD

Constantly alternate a game of catch, whereby the tagged player must always keep one of his hands on the place where he was touched. If he touches another player as the catcher, he is able to move freelyagain. Depending on the chosen group size, multiple players can be designated catchers. Field size should be determined based on the training and teaching goal.

See how often you were touched within a specific period of time.

EXERCISE 11: TORTURE

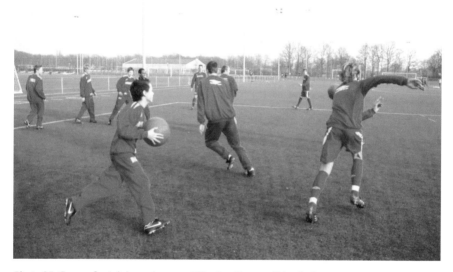

Photo 25: Game of catch is made more difficult with a medicine ball.

Constantly alternate a game of catch, whereby the catcher must also carry a medicine ball. He can only touch a player with his free hand. Depending on the chosen group size, multiple players can be designated catchers. Field size should be determined based on the training and teaching goal (e.g., 15 x 15 m).

See how often you were touched within a specified time period.

EXERCISE 12: CAUTION, CONSTRUCTION ZONE!

Constantly alternate a game of catch, whereby benches (medicine balls, hurdles or mini hurdles, or agility ladders) that the catcher is not allowed to run or jump over are placed on the marked playing field.

Depending on the chosen group size, multiple players can be designated catchers. Field size should be determined based on the training and teaching goal.

See how often you were touched within a specified time period.

EXERCISE 13: DIVERSION

Constantly alternate a game of catch, whereby a third player is allowed to sprint between the catcher and the hunted without getting touched. If he succeeds, the catcher must try to catch this player.

Depending on the chosen group size, multiple players can be designated catchers. Field size should be determined based on the training and teaching goal.

See how often you were touched within a specified time period.

See who helps the hunted with a diversion maneuver. It requires teamwork.

EXERCISE 14: TEAMWORK

Four catchers each have a baton or wooden staff. Together the four catchers try to continuously touch two players. If they succeed, the second of the two tagged players receives a baton or wooden staff. The catchers continue until they have given away all of the batons or staffs.

a) What is the total time for all four players?

b) Who was touched during a specified time period or not at all?

Field size should be determined based on the training and teaching goal.

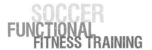

9.2.2   FORMS OF TEAMWORK – CATCHING GAMES

By now there is lots of empirical evidence from sports science research, unequivocally documenting that implicit and explicit processes of appropriation in games function autonomously and simultaneously in cooperating or competing interaction. Collective action structures that are a part of the complex game of soccer also develop in the form of unconscious but (highly) intelligent cognitive processes so that, for instance, requirements considered difficult (e.g., enormous competitive stress and new and difficult tasks) can be met by the player with precision, speed, versatility, as well as situationally in forms of play.

The authors are, therefore, of the opinion that the important aspect of teamwork should already be stressed during introductory games of catch. It should be understood and practiced from the perspective of the catchers as well as the hunted.

EXERCISE 1: SIAMESE TWINS

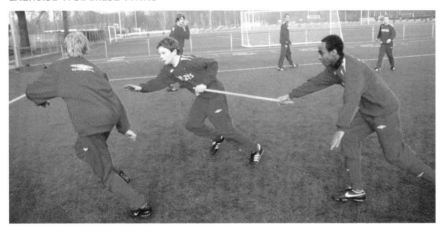

Photo 26: Cutting off the running lane together.

Two players link hands, or as shown in photo 26, each hold the end of a stick. Their task is to touch as many players as possible within a specific time period.

Depending on the chosen group size, multiple pairs can be designated. Field size is usually 15 x 15 meters.

VARIATIONS:

- Jump ropes, Thera-Bands, Vario bands, or tubes with handles can also be used for pairing up.
- Once a teammate has been touched, he takes over that place in the pair.
- Choose two fields that take up the size of a volleyball court. There is one pair of catchers in each field. Each pair tries to touch as many players as possible within their field. Each tagged player must immediately switch to the other field and continue play there.
- Group size and playing time depend on the training and teaching goal. See which of the two pairs can keep their field clear for a specified time period.
- Form a group of three with two sticks. This creates a chain of three in which the middle player has the task of coordinator since he is unable to touch players while holding both sticks. He decides and controls the running lanes and actions. Group size and playing time depend on the training and teaching goal. See how often the individual players have to switch fields.

EXERCISE 2: BEWARE OF DOG!

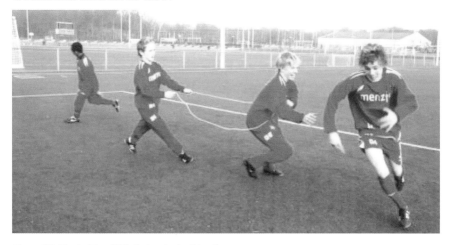

Photo 27: The holder skillfully leads the "dog."

Two players, linked by a rope, work together as dog and dog holder. The rope is tied around the dog's waist, and the holder steers him in the direction of the players he needs to catch on the playing field.

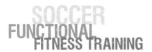

Field size, group size, and playing time depend on the training and teaching goal. (In photo 27, it is 15 x 15 m.)

Choose rules of the game based on the first form.

VARIATION:

◉ Same as before—the hunted players also pair up.

EXERCISE 3: CHAIN OF THREE

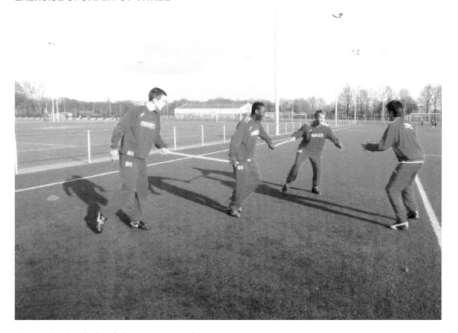

Photo 28: The chain of three corners a player.

Compare to exercise 2 variation, whereby the player who was touched trades places with the middle player in the chain of three. The player in the chain of three who executed the touch is now able to move freely around the field. Field size, group size, and playing time depend on the training and teaching goal. (In photo 28, it is 15 x 15 m.) Choose rules of the game based on the first form.

See who was never touched. These players can become the catchers in the chain of three during subsequent rounds.

EXERCISE 4: CATCHING CHAINS

The game starts with one catcher. He and the player he touches then form a pair of catchers. Each additional tagged player joins them, forming a chain. Only the outside players in the chain can touch players. Running under the chain is permitted.

Field size, group size, and playing time depend on the training and teaching goal.

See who is left in the end.

VARIATION:

◉ Start with two catchers so that two chains form.

EXERCISE 5: OCTOPUS

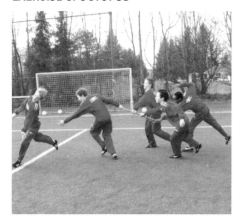

Photo 29: Four players holding on to a stick form an octopus.

A pair of catchers are linked by a stick. When a player is touched, he has to hold on to the stick. If another player is touched, he must also hold on to the stick so that an octopus forms (see photo 29). When the most outside player touches someone, that player must hold on to the middle of the stick. Each additional player that is touched must trade places with the player who touched him. Starting with two pairs of catchers has proven successful in practice.

Field size, group size, and playing time depend on the training and teaching goal. (In photo 29, it is 15 x 15 m.)

See who was rarely the octopus.

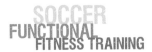
EXERCISE 6: LEAPFROG

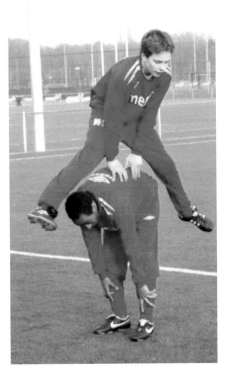

Game of catch with two catchers, whereby each tagged player must get in a crouch position. The free players can "release" him by leapfrogging over him.

Field size, group size, and playing time depend on the training and teaching goal.

POSSIBLE RULES:

a) See how many players are left in a crouch position.

b) See who was in a crouch least often.

c) See how often you were in a crouch position.

d) See who released the most players.

Photo 30: Who can "release" the crouching player with teamwork?

EXERCISE 7: TUNNELING

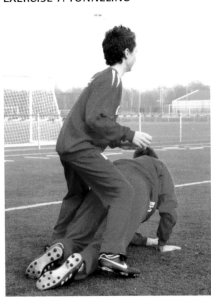

Execution and rules of the game are the same as exercise 6, whereby the player who has been touched must stand in a straddle position so a teammate can crawl (tunnel) through his legs, and in doing so, "release" him. Field size is generally 15 x 15 meters.

It is recommended to use multiple catchers.

Photo 31: Dexterity is key!

EXERCISE 8: TICKING

The catchers can only touch someone who isn't holding a ball, stick, cone, bib, or something similar in his hands. To create changing situations in which the teammates have to help each other, the following rule can be enacted: When a player receives one of the previously mentioned objects from a teammate, no one can touch him. Having 50% of players with objects and 50% without has proven successful in practice. When a player has been touched, he can continue to play. The number of catchers is based on the group size. Field size, group size, and playing time depend on the training and teaching goal.

RULE OF THE GAME:

See who has touched the most players within a specified time period.

VARIATION:

❯ Players can only touch someone who is holding a ball or other object in his hands.

EXERCISE 9: ESCAPE AGENT

Create a game of catch in which the tagged players must wait at a cone or hoop. The coach or instructor chooses one or two players who can release these players by touching them in the course of the game. The tagged players can also form a chain with other players in one spot so the entire group can be released by the touch of one player (at the chain ends). Field size, group size, and playing time depend on the training/teaching goal.

RULE OF THE GAME:

❯ See who has released the most players within a specified time period.

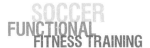

EXERCISE 10: PARCOURS

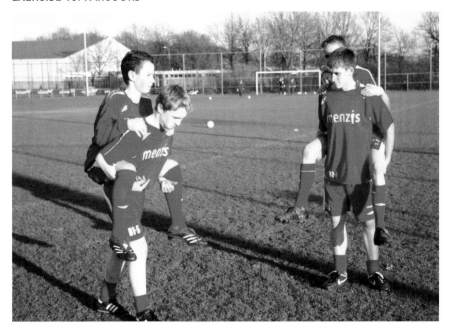

Photo 32: A secure position requires strength and teamwork.

Start a game of catch on a field marked 15 x 15 meters, whereby two players work together. The teammates must try to protect themselves from the catcher by quickly "piggybacking" onto another player's back. Players who are "piggybacking" on someone else's back or chest cannot be touched. Motto: Everyone helps everyone else by piggybacking and carrying. You are not allowed to

a) choose the same player twice in a row, or

b) change partner positions on the spot.

Field size, group size, and playing time depend on the training and teaching goal.

RULE OF THE GAME:

❯ See who has touched the most players within a specified period of time.

EXERCISE 11: FIELD CHANGE

Divide a large field into two smaller fields. There are two catchers in each half. Two catchers have a ball (possibly even a medicine ball). The catchers try to touch the players in both halves with the ball. This is not done by throwing the ball but rather by firmly pressing the ball into the teammate who is sprinting away. Since the catchers have only one ball, they must cooperate and communicate. Once a player has been tagged with the ball, he must switch to the other field where he can continue to play. Field size, group size, and playing time depend on the training and teaching goal

RULES OF THE GAME:

a) See which of the two pairs of catchers has the fewest number of players in their half during a specified time period.

b) See how often the players who run away have to switch fields.

VARIATION:

❯ Four players in each field are marked with colored bibs. Each field also has a small group of players in possession of a ball. The catchers are not allowed to run with the ball. Once a player has been touched with the ball he must switch to the other field, where he can continue to play.

RULE OF THE GAME:

❯ See which team with a ball has the fewest running players in its field. Regularly alternate tasks.

EXERCISE 12: QUICK CHECKER

Two teams play against each other on one field. One team has ball possession. This team must try to touch players on the other team through cooperation and communication. But players cannot run with the ball. Passing trumps. When a player has been tagged, players immediately change roles. Field size, group size, and playing time depend on the training and teaching goal

RULE OF THE GAME:

❯ See which team successfully avoids being tagged the longest. Coach or instructor keeps the time.

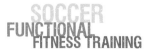

VARIATION:

◈ Do the same variation as in exercise 2 in which each team has a ball.

RULE OF THE GAME:

◈ See which team is quickest to tag the opposing team without getting tagged themselves. Coach or instructor keeps the time.

9.2.3   SKILLFULLY OVERCOMING OBSTACLES – CATCHING GAMES

Dribbling around, outplaying, and running around the opponent and properly tackling with physical contact play a major role in soccer. Catching games are a good way to address these situations. But the coach or instructor must make sure thatcompetition rules are observed—don't tolerate deliberate rule violations, such as blocking or pushing.

Motto: As little physical contact as possible, as much physical contact as necessary.

EXERCISE 1: FLAGS

Each player has a bib, visible and easy to grasp, tucked into his waistband. It's all against all with the following rules:

Players try to capture and collect their teammates' bibs. If a player loseshis own bib he can get another one from the coach or instructor and continue to play. Field size, group size, and playing time depend on the training and teaching goal.

RULE OF THE GAME:

◈ See who has collected the most bibs within a specified time period.

VARIATION:

◈ Two teams with different color bibs play against each other.

RULE OF THE GAME:

◈ See which group collects the most bibs within a specified period of time.

EXERCISE 2: WANDERING CIRCLE

Form circles with five players in each. After a signal from the coach, another player tries to touch the back of one of the players in the circle.

Field size and playing time depend on the training and teaching goal.

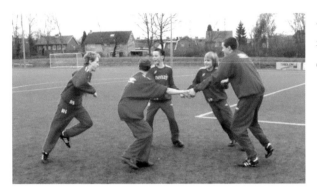

Photo 33: Hold on tight and stay together to evade the attacker.

RULE OF THE GAME:

- See who touches one of the players in the circle in the least amount of time. Coach or instructor keeps the time.

EXERCISE 3: SAFETY FIRST

The attacker (catcher) tries to touch the back of the last player in the line. By using their arms and skillful forward, backward, and sideways movements, the players can delay the catcher by 10 to 15 seconds. Holding and pushing are not allowed. Coordinated teamwork relative to one's position in the line is absolutely necessary.

Field size and group size depend on the training and teaching goal.

The coach or instructor keeps the time.

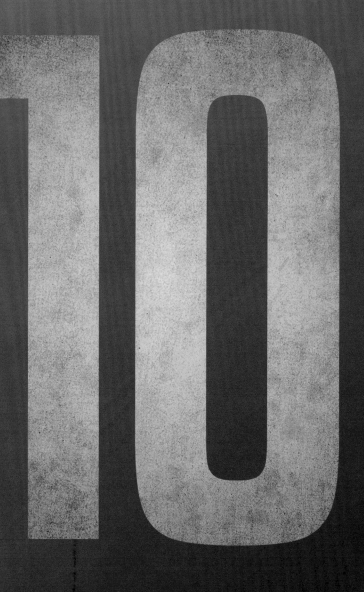

CHAPTER

10

10 RUNNING GAMES WITHOUT A BALL

> *"In the soccer learning process, lack of time is the biggest enemy."*

(van Lingen and Pauw, 1999/2000, p. 227)

Many of the catching games in chapter 9 can be considered running games. But the difference lies in the objectives. The catching games we introduced are used for preparation (warm-up) to create a relaxed, joyous, and focused training atmosphere. They are also used to introduce the educational aspect of cooperation andthe use of basic coordination abilities and physical performance factors. They should form the basis for the specialization process in continuing soccer training.

In this chapter, the authors will focus on running games.

10.1 CHASING GAMES

All team players sit together in a circle. The coach or instructor passes out numbers 1 through 4. Field size, group size, and playing time depend on the training and teaching goal.

RULES OF THE GAME:
- The coach or instructor calls out one of the numbers. All players with that number run clockwise or counterclockwise (specify direction) and try to touch the player in front of them. Anyone who is tagged returns to his seat (through the circle). While the players run or sprint, the coach can shout "reverse," and the players quickly change direction and partners.

VARIATION:
- Everyone with the number called runs the number of rounds previously specified by the coach. Please pass on the outside! See who is the first one back to his seat.

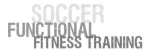

10.2 CHANGE OF LOCATION

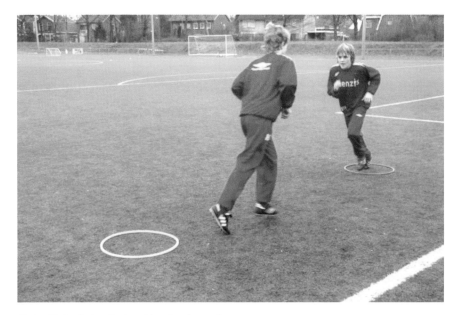

Photo 35: Explosive start and leaning forward

The players spread out on a marked playing field. They position themselves inside a hoop or next to a bar, cone, or mat. On the field there are two controllers who try to take over (occupy) a base whenever the players change locations. When they succeed, the controller becomes a player, and vice versa.

Field size, group size, and playing time depend on the training and teaching goal. (In photo 35, the field is 15 x 15 meters.)

RULES OF THE GAME:

- Trading places with the same teammate twice is not allowed. See who can change locations the most.

10.3 BASES

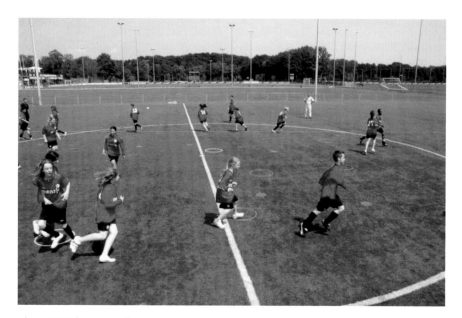

Photo 36: Being successful, even in chaos!

Six mats, hoops, large dots, or other items are spread around the playing field.

Field size, group size, and playing time depend on the training and teaching goal. (In photo 36, they are in the center circle on a big field.)

RULES OF THE GAME:

- Choose two players who will try to prevent players from claiming hoops.Players claim hoops by touching them. Each hoop claimed earns one bonus point. Each touch results in tasks being switched: The player becomes the hunter, but keeps the bonus points he has earned until the next switch. He is not allowed to try to capture the same hoop twice. If a player stays inside the hoop, he cannot be touched.
- See who scores the most bonus points.

VARIATION:

- Running game for two.

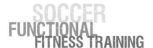
10.4 ROLLERCOASTER

The team forms a rollercoaster and takes up a permanent position. The coach or instructor chooses a player who runs clockwise around the rollercoaster and touches no more than four players. The size of the rollercoaster, the team, and length of running time depend on the training and teaching goal.

RULES OF THE GAME:

- All players first adopt the pace of the individual player and, after a signal from the coach, must try to return to their old positions.
- See who is the fastest player in the rollercoaster.

10.5 SPEED TRAIN

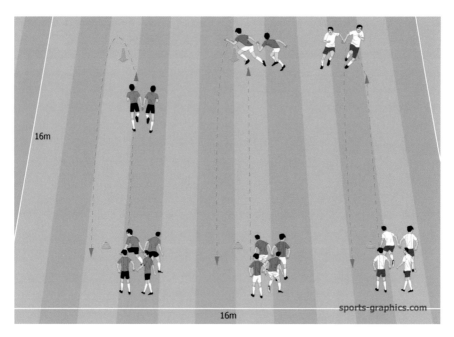

Fig. 8: The train "grows" in pairs!

As shown in fig. 8, the first pairs start by running around the cones and back with their hands linked. Next they take the second pair along with them, continuing until all pairs are part of the train. The distance between cones, team size, and number of repetitions depend on the training and teaching goal. (In fig. 8, the field is 16 x 16 meters.)

RULES OF THE GAME:

- If the players lose hand contact, the train must stop and can only accelerate again once all handcontact has been reestablished.
- See which speed train is the first to return to the starting point with all its cars.

VARIATIONS:

1. First the train accelerates with all the "cars" and then loses one car (pair) after each round. Please specify the order within the teams first.
2. Now combine the original rule and the first variation.

10.6 PAINTBALL

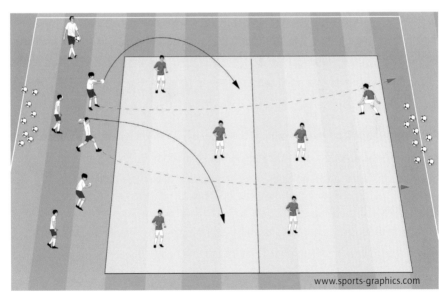

www.sports-graphics.com

Fig. 9: Sprinting, looking, and reacting

The blue team (see fig. 9) gets in position and throws one or two softballs into one of the two fields. Next all blue players try to get to the other side without being tagged by one of the two red team balls (see fig. 9). Red can use the balls directly or indirectly (with ground contact) against the players. Throws to the head should be avoided.

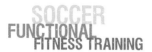
Field size, team size (6-on-6 in fig. 9), and the number of repetitions depend on the training and teaching goal.

RULES OF THE GAME:

- See how many times a group of runners manages to switch sides without getting tagged by the ball.Coach or instructor counts the number of runs.

VARIATIONS:

1. The coach or instructor issues a time allowance depending on the training goal. See which team gets the fewest hits within the time allowed.
2. Same setup as the game, using various additional items placed on the fields: dummies, mini goals, benches, or cones. Additional balls can also be used.

10.7 MIMICRY

Teams of four to five players line up in a row. Each player on a team gets a number. Players with the number one perform certain movements (e.g., running, skipping, running backward, walking fast, single-leg jumps, jumpingjacks). His teammates mimic his movements to a predetermined point. Next it is the turn of the player with the number two, and so on.

Field size, team size (here, four to five players), and the number of repetitions depend on the training and teaching goal. Please pay particular attention to an adequate distance between teams to decrease the risk of colliding.

VARIATION:

- Form groups of two, facing each other. One player is the leader, and the other player mimics him. Creativity and variety are needed here!

10.8 SUPER SPRINT

Two players face each other 10 meters apart. A cone or something similar is placed between the two players. One of the two players (A) must take the initiative and run to the cone, trying to pick it up before returning to his starting point.

RULES OF THE GAME:

- ◈ On his way to the cone he must imitate movements that can occur in a soccer game, such as sidestepping, turning, and jumping. His teammate (B) must imitate him. When player A picks up the cone, player B must try to tag him before player A can return to his starting point (finish line). Then they switch tasks. Pease make sure to plan for asufficient amount of space between the pairs.

- ◈ The number of repetitions and the break lengths depend on the training and teaching goal.

10.9 SOCCER QUIZ

Mark three fields, or circles, at equal distances around the team. Each field is assigned a task: Field 1 is soccer superstars; field 2 is first to third division Bundesliga teams; field 3 is Champions League teams. Initially players can move about freely.

RULES OF THE GAME:

- ◈ The coach or instructor calls out a familiar term, such as Messi. The players must then sprint as fast as possible into field 1. The last player to reach field 1 gets a penalty point, but can still participate.

- ◈ See which player can finish the soccer quiz without getting a penalty point.

- ◈ The distance to the fields, number of repetitions, and break lengths depend on the training and teaching goal.

VARIATIONS:

1. Players dribble or juggle during breaks and then sprint on command.
2. The coach or instructor calls out up to three terms in a row.
3. Two groups: Group 1 is with the head coach or instructor; group 2 is with the assistant coach or class representative. Both perform the soccer quiz with their groups at the same time. Remind the players that concentration is required.

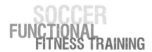

10.10 THE MISSION

Mark a circle and assign each player a permanent spot. It can be marked with a hoop, mat, or cone. In addition, items are placed at equal distances (outside and inside) that are associated with a certain task, provided next.

RULES OF THE GAME:
- Carry out the mission assigned by the coach or instructor and immediately return to your spot. The last player gets a penalty point, but can still participate. See which player manages to finish the mission game without getting a penalty point.
- The distance to the items, the size of the circle, the number of repetitions, and the break lengths depend on the training and teaching goal.

POSSIBLE MISSIONS:
1. Touch four cones located inside the circle and sprint back to your spot.
2. First run around the poles placed far outside the circle and then sprint back to your spot.

Remind players to watch out for their teammates to decrease the risk of colliding.

10.11 SPEED KING

Use the same setup as 10.10, but this time the players must run up to items inside and outside the circle and touch them with a part of their body and then remain there.

RULES OF THE GAME:
- At the coach's or instructor's command (e.g., "Pole"), the players sprint toward that item. It is important that there are fewer items than the total number of players. Players who are unable to reach an item in time get a penalty point and continue to play. After each task, the coach or instructor removes one item, so there are fewer and fewer "open places" for all players. The game ends and a new one starts when approximately one-third of players are unable to find an open spot.
- See which player or players get the fewest penalty points.

❱ The distance to the items, the size of the circle, the number of repetitions, and the break lengths depend on the training and teaching goal. Remind players to watch out for their teammates to decrease the risk of colliding.

VARIATION:

❱ The coach or instructor says a number. The players must run to the given number of items (e.g., benches, hoops, cones) and touch them, reamining at the final item. If unsuccessful, the player or players get a penalty point. See who is able to get the fewest penalty points in10 races, for example.

10.12 ORBIT

The team forms two circles, one inner and one outer. Each player has a partner; for example, player A is in the inner circle, and his teammate, player B, is in the outer circle. At a signal from the coach or instructor, the circles move in opposite directions. Players must try to keep their running speed and distances to each other consistent.

RULES OF THE GAME:

❱ At a signal from the coach or instructor (e.g., whistle or clap), the pairs find each other and one player piggybacks onto the other. The last pair to complete this task gets a penalty point, but can continue to participate.

❱ The size of the circles, the number of repetitions, and the break lengths depend on the training and teaching goal. Remind players to watch out for your teammates to decrease the risk of colliding.

VARIATION:

❱ Open choice of partner: See which pair is the last to get in piggyback position.

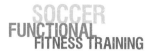
10.13 THE CLOCK IS RUNNING

Spread six hoops around a marked field. The coach or instructor designates two catchers.

RULES OF THE GAME:

- Each player on the team must touch as many hoops as possible in 30 seconds. He can also stop inside a hoop. The players are not allowed to run back and forth between two hoops, and the catchers cannot wait for a player in front of a hoop. If the player is tagged before he can reach his hoops, he gets a penalty point, but can continue to participate. Regularly alternate catchers.

- See who is able to run to the most hoops in 30 seconds.

- Field size, the distances between hoops, the duration, the number of hoops, the number of repetitions, and the break lengths depend on the training and teaching goal. Remind players to watch out for their teammates to decrease the risk of colliding.

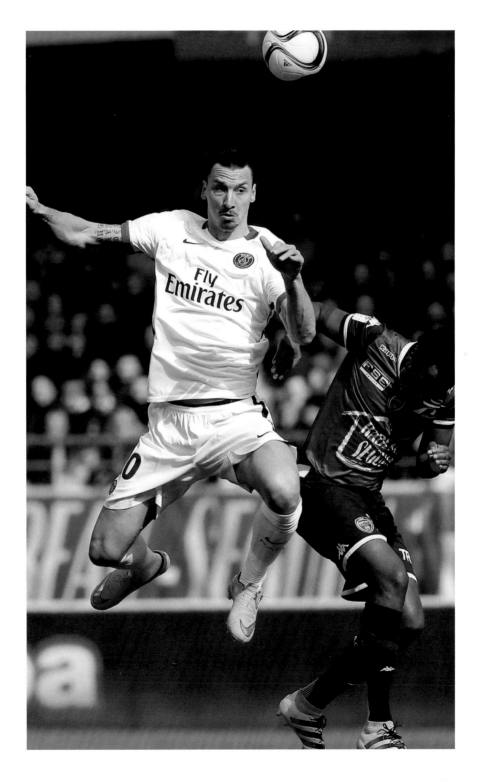

> CHAPTER

11

11 RUNNING GAMES WITH A BALL

> *"The ball sets the pace. There has never been a soccer player who was faster than the ball."*

(Johan Cruyff quoted in Verheijen, 1999/2000, p. 182)

Running games in soccer practice (see chapter 10) can be easily combined with target practice games, end zone games, and sport-related ball games. In due consideration of the modules **feel for the ball, pressure of time, pressure of precision, pressure of complexity, organizational pressure, pressure of variability and stress,** they are particularly wellsuited for teaching cognitive skills, information processing, attention span, and creativity. They are used in warm-ups, as follow-ups to and preparation for coordination training, basic proficiency-related skills (e.g., recognizing the opponent or obstacle), and the basic tactical competencies (e.g., cooperatively safeguarding possession) with a view to ball training and cool-down. Their stimulating nature with the ball generates a largely joyful training atmosphere with beginners as well as pro players and with respect to coaching, teambuilding (educational perspective), and active relaxation, represents a not to be underestimated instrument for training management.

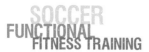

EXERCISE 1: RUNNER AGAINST PASSING PLAYER

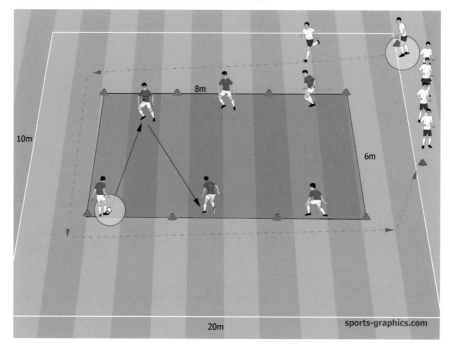

Fig. 10: 90-degree turns at top speed versus triangle passing

One after another, the runners (white team) must complete a marked course. In the meantime, the red team passes the ball back and forth on the small field.

RULES OF THE GAME:

- The passing players pass the ball back and forth for as long as the runners are running. Each pass is counted. As soon as all runners have crossed the finish line, everyone switches. See which team was able to make the most passes.

- The length of the running school, the size of the small field, the number of runners and passers, and repetitions depend on the training goal.

VARIATION:

- Form 1.1: Sprinting and turning and forward passes. Field sizes are as shown in fig. 10.

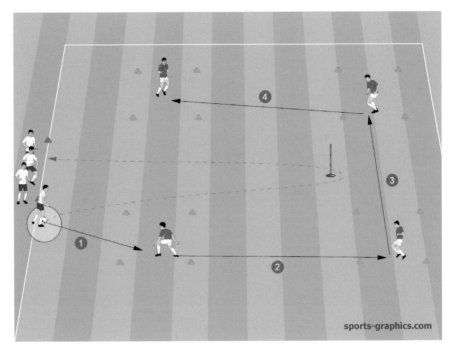

Fig. 11: 180-degree turn at top speed versus precise forward passes

Set up the same as form 1.1, plus 18 cones and a pole in which the angle and length ratios differ between running and passing. Use caution when playing a forward pass diagonally to the running direction.

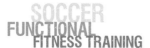

EXERCISE 2: HOT ZONE

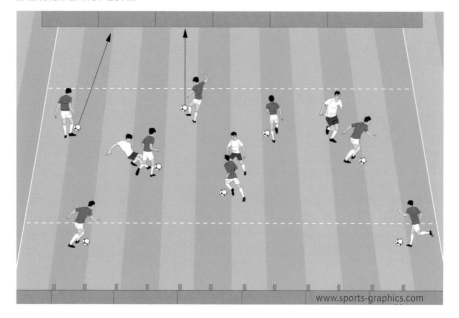

Fig. 12: Fast dribbles and duels through "battle players"

The object is to cross the hot zone (zone between the two broken lines) with the ball as many times as possible within a specific time period and shoot on the goals in the cool space (in fig. 12, overturned benches). But there are battle players in the hot zone —in fig. 12, three white players—who will try to separate the players from the ball by

- ❂   seeking out duels and passing won balls on;
- ❂   preventing passes in direction of the goal by tackling; and
- ❂   clearing a ball that rolls toward the goal.

Players, the eight in red, can only score from the hot zone. Balls that stop between the goals and the hot zone or end up out of play can be dribbled back into the hot zone unchallenged by the eight players. At no time can the hands come in contact with the ball.

RULES OF THE GAME:

- Each player has a ball. A player scores a point every time he manages to successfully get through the hot zone and scores a goal. See which red player scores the most goals. Alternate regularly.

- Field size, size of hot zones, number of players, battle players, the amount of time for a round, break lengths, and number of repetitions depend on the training goal.

EXERCISE 3: SIAMESE SOCCER

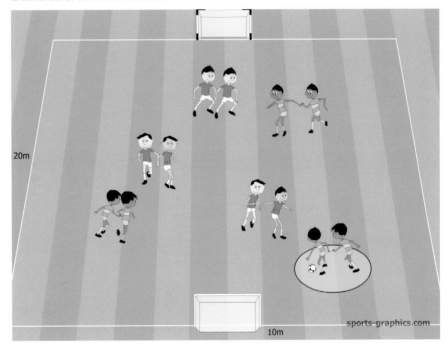

Fig. 13: Cooperation is required.

Two players always link hands and as a pair try to score a goal in the opposing half.

RULES OF THE GAME:

- Pairs must keep hands linked while running, dribbling, passing, and shooting. There can be no contact between hands and ball. When a goal is scored, the opposing pairs fall back into their half of the field so a calm buildup can take place.

- Field size, number of pairs, duration, and break lengths depend on the training goal (10 x 20 m in fig. 3).

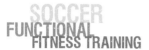

EXERCISE 4: SOCCER-BURNING BALL

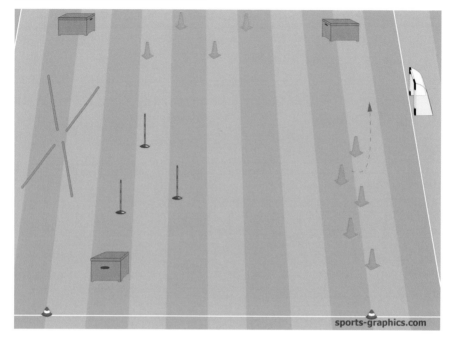

Fig. 14: Lots of equipment is used here with a minigoal as the burn (base).

A combination of burning ball and soccer, meaning the team of runners brings the ball into the game, and the team on the field takes the ball and tries to pass or shoot it as quickly as possible into the burn (base).

RULES OF THE GAME:

- The first player from the team of runners kicks the ball onto the field. The field players must play the ball as quickly as possible to the burn (mini goal). To do so, they must play through three open goals built from small boxes, poles, and cones. At the same time, the team of runners tries to play a second ball once around the field. To do so, they must dribble around the slalom poles and negotiate tight spots. Each player gets three points if he can make it to the finish line without a break, otherwise just one point. If a player is caught between the open goals (meaning the other team plays the first ball into the mini goal before he can finish his run), he goes directly to the finish, but does not score a point.

- Field size (16 x 16 m in fig. 14), number of players per team, duration, number of repetitions, and the equipment used depend on the training goal.

EXERCISE 5: AMERICAN SPEEDBALL

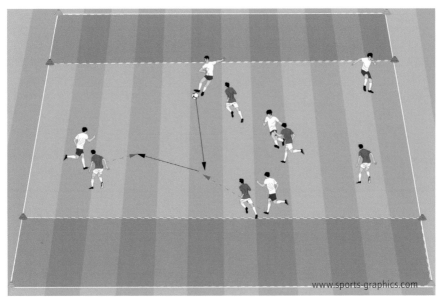

Fig. 15: Passing with hand and foot

Similar to rugby, the ball (soccer ball or futsal) is passed into the opposing end zone using passes and runs.

RULES OF THE GAME:

❂ The game opens with a kick from the own end line. As soon as the opposing team has settled the ball they can start an attack according to soccer rules. If a pass is caught (with the foot), the player can keep running with the ball. There is no step limit. If the ball is caught directly from the air after a pass in the opposing end zone, the team is awarded two points. A run into the end zone earns the team three points. As long as the ball doesn't touch the ground, it can also be passed by hand. The player who catches the ball can keep running with the ball. The defending team is allowed to intercept passes. With a quick transition they can launch their own attack. If the player carrying the ball is tagged on the back by a defender, the run stops, and the ball changes possession. The game is then started over with the foot.

❂ Field size, size of end zones, number of players per team, and the duration of the runs depend on the training goal.

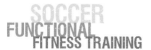

EXERCISE 6: SCUFFLE BALL

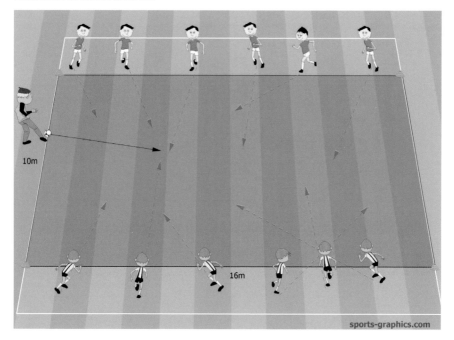

Fig. 16a: Fair play in spite of a physical game. No fear of physical contact!

In this game the players must use powerful acceleration speed to move the ball beyond the opposing line.

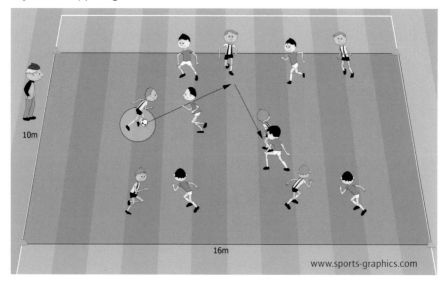

Fig. 16b

RULES OF THE GAME:

- A drop ball starts the game in the center of the field. At the beginning, the remaining players from the two teams spread out in the two target areas— the light-green areas of the two head sides (end zones)—and after the drop ball they move into the inner playing field (darkgreen). A point is scored when the ball is dribbled into the respective end zone and is stopped there. The ball can be dribbled in any direction.

- Passes can only be played to the rear. The defending team cannot enter their end zone to defend. They must try to get possession through the proper means: pressing, tackling, bumping, shielding the ball with the body. Only the player in possession can be attacked directly. After each point scored, the game starts over with a drop ball.

- The player with the ball can be stopped with a slight tag on the back. If this happens, he must immediately pass the ball to a teammate behind him. The tagged player then runs back to his own zone and can once again participate in the action. The tagged player must stop the ball (the ball must be at rest), and the tagger plays it on. Rule violations like unfair and rough play result in turnovers or time penalties. The coach or instructor acts as referee.

- The ball (e.g., soccer ball, futsal, tennis ball), field size (inside area approximately 10 x 16 m in fig.16a-c), size of the end zones, number of players per team, and duration of the rounds depend on the training goals.

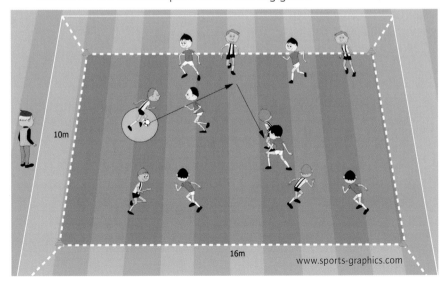

10m

16m

www.sports-graphics.com

Fig. 16c

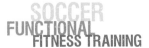
EXERCISE 7: TEAM BALL

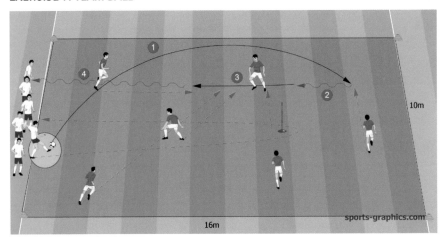

10m

16m

sports-graphics.com

Fig. 17: Which team can get organized quickest?

The blue team kicks the ball onto the field and runs around a pole and back to the starting point (baseline). The red team catches or receives the ball and together forms a tunnel at the receiving point. The last man passes the ball between the other players' legs to the front man, who dribbles it behind the baseline. At the same time he shouts, "Team!" Any of the runners who have not reached the baseline at that time get a penalty point.

RULES OF THE GAME:

- See how many runners were able to reach the line before the shout and how many penalty points the runners accumulated. If the runners on the blue team are faster than the red team, the team is awarded bonus points in the amount of the number of players on that team. Regularly alternate tasks and check the score after a predetermined number of rounds between blue versus red.See which team has the fewest penalty points.

- The ball (e.g., soccer ball, futsal, tennis ball), field size (10 x 16 m in fig. 17), distance from baseline to turning point (pole), number of players per team, and duration of the rounds depend on the training goals.

EXERCISE 8: STRESS BALL

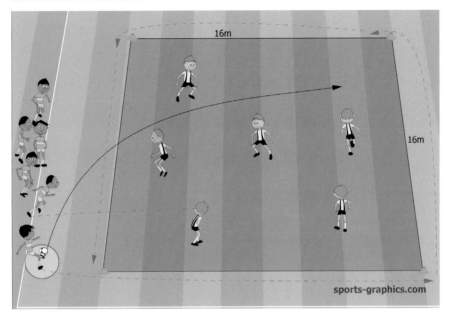

Fig. 18: Cooperation, speed, and dexterity

After kicking a ball onto the field, one runner from the running team tries to run a predetermined distance to score a point. The field teammust try to prevent him from doing so.

RULES OF THE GAME:

- One of the runners plays a volley onto the field and right after tries to run around the field.

- Another member of the running team (green/yellow) runs onto the opposing field. If he manages not to get shot down until his teammate has rounded the four cones, his team scores a point.

- After runners and field players switch roles, the scores are compared at the end of the game.

- Soft foam balls, field size (16 x 16 m in fig. 18), number of players per team, and number of rounds depend on the training goal.

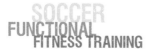

EXERCISE 9: KEEPER'STCHOUKBALL GAME

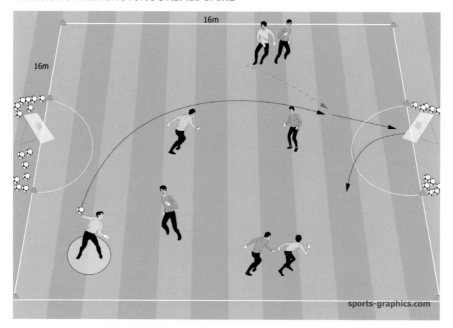

Fig. 19: Throwing, running, jumping, and catching

The premise of throwing a ball toward a target in such a way that the opposing team has trouble receiving the rebounding ball stems from the Spanish game of Pelota.

RULES OF THE GAME:

- A point is scored whenever the attacking team throws the ball onto the frame (the target area is a kind of miniature trampoline) or volleysor shoots it so that it touches the ground on the playing field before a defending keeper (here blue/black) can catch it. The keepers are not allowed to illegally hamper each other during the catching attempts. The goal box cannot be entered during the throw on goal or defensive play. A ball that bounces off the frame and lands in the goal box is invalid. Opposing keepers are not allowed to intercept the ball. The ball must be thrown at the frame after no more then three passes.

- A soccer ball and (replacement balls), the size of the field (16 x 16 m in fig. 19) and the goal box, the number of keepers per team, and the playing time depend on the training goal.

EXERCISE 10: INDIRECT MAT BALL FOR THE KEEPER

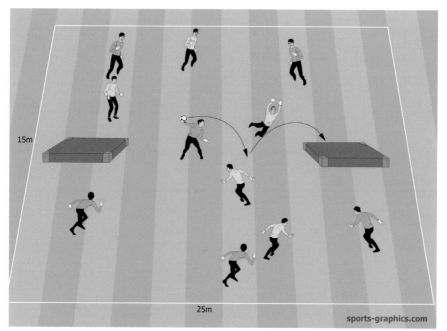

Fig. 20: Passing and catching for the keeper

The game's objective is to hit a mat with the ball using an indirect throw to the ground or to prevent the ball from hitting the mat.

RULES OF THE GAME:

- The ball is played with the hand or as a volley with the foot (also called lob pass). The defending keepers can dive for and fend off the rebounding ball (during a throw in direction of the opposing mat) above the soft floor mat. Only one to two steps can be taken with the ball. Dribbling the ball is not allowed. See which team scores the most mat hits.
- A soccer ball and replacement balls, the size of the field and the soft floor mat, the number of keepers per team, and the playing time depend on the training goal.

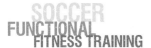

EXERCISE 11: SEPAKTAKRAW

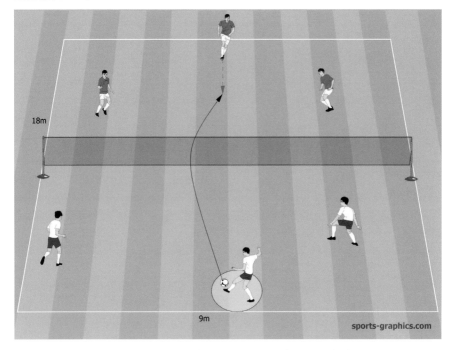

Fig. 21: This Asian game promotes dexterity, cooperation, and communication.

A game that harkens back to very old traditions all over Asia, it centers on a ball woven from rattan.

RULES OF THE GAME:

- Three players on one team play the ball over the net in such a way that it hopefully hits the ground on the opponent's side. The ball is played over the net from the hands to the foot and caught the same way. Before catching the ball, it must be touched with the chest, upper thigh, or head. The player can no longer pass the ball forward; rather, it must be served by another player. The ball should no longer be caught or thrown, but as in footballtennis, it can bounce one time.

- See which team scores the most points.

- A ball woven from rattan or another kind of ball with similar properties, field size (9 x 18 m in fig. 21), the height of the net or the cord, the number of players per team, and the playing time depend on the training goal.

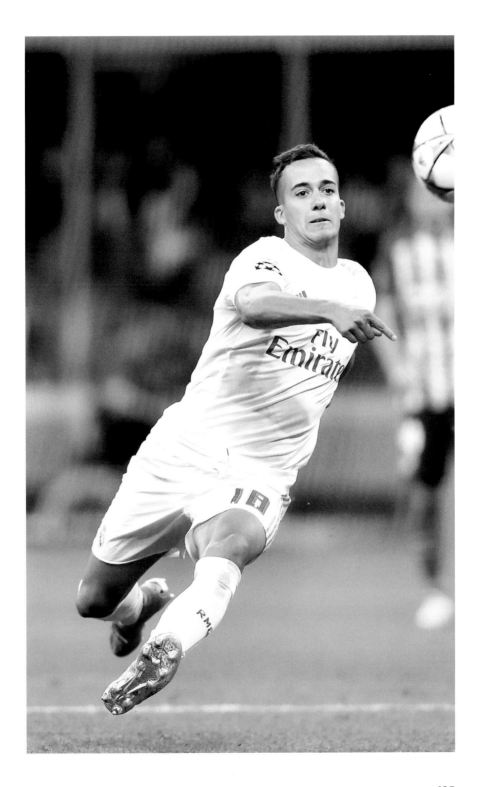

> CHAPTER

12

12 LITTLE RUNNING SCHOOL FOR SOCCER PLAYERS

"An improved running technique does not only result in a higher maximum running speed, but also facilitates more economical running at slower speeds."

(Dr. W. Schöllhorn, 2003, p. 8)

A running school for soccer payers is a useful addition to the running games played with and without the ball. In the authors' opinion, the coach or instructor should possess the basic running knowledge that will be showcased in this chapter, with the goal of creating a customized range of forms for his training.[20]

A running posture that can greatly interfere with a soccer player's ability to run fast is exhibited in photos 37 and 38.

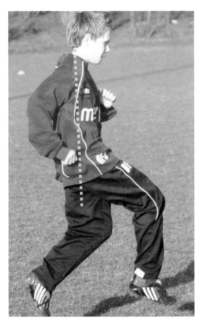

Photo 37: "Not like that!" This youth player "sits" while he runs. The proof is in the broken line acrosshisbody alignment.

---

20   *Additional information on kinetics can be found in Schöllhorn, 2003.)*

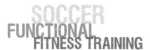
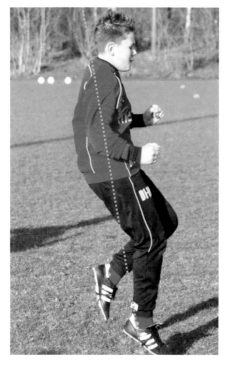

Photo 38: "And not like that either!" This player does a countermotion with his arms and "hikes" his trunk and shoulders up and leans back while running, as shown by the broken line.

Which goals can a coach or instructor pursue with a running school for soccer players?

- Improving generalrunning fitness
- Improving running technique, such as footstrike, knee and hip extension, and head, trunk, and arm position[21]
- Increasing length and frequency of passes with respect to running motions
- Improving starting speed
- Developing a sense of timing and tempo
- Doing tempo runs, whereby the speed gradually increases in the course of a previously specified distance until 100% of the maximum speed is reached; here the coach or instructor pays close attention to technical aspects of running that must be more closelydefined

---

21   *Interested readers can find additional relevant information on the development of the short sprint in Buckwitz and Stein (2014, p. 42-44). They ascribe the performance explosion in the men's 100-meter sprint to the following criterion: An increase in maximum speed due to a longer acceleration phase and concomitant implementation of a longer stride. This fact can be of great interest in soccer training because with high lines (and consequently larger spaces behind the last line of defense), active chains of three with larger spaces (during turnovers from offensive pressing) for opposing passes into seams, and more wing play, the number of short sprints without the ball will continue to increase. In youth soccer we can often see that a short stride, particularly at the beginning, with short sprints into open space is favored and even practiced. The support phase continues to be of major importance in the short sprints of world-class runners. For soccer training, particularly in high-performance soccer, these findings may indicate a future increase in selective training of the ischiocrural muscles for acceleration and the quadriceps for touchdown stress. The authors recommend shorter tempo runs, speed chutes, and downhill runs, and selective weight training for hip flexors and extensors through isokinetic strength training equipment and the well-known sprint strength training apparatus by Tidow. From a technical standpoint, a pronounced front support should be avoided, and instead emphasis should be placed on a high knee lift, with the goal of achieving major acceleration of the foot towards the ground (see p. 42-43; see also chapter 17.2).*

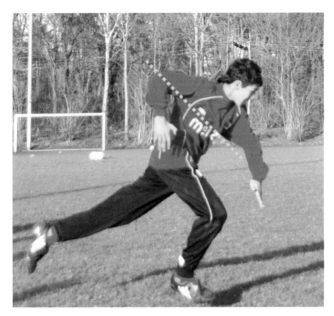

A running school can be held in the gym, a park, or at the soccer park. It is the authors' opinion that the running school should not exceed the following durations and training loads for age groups 15 and younger.

Photo 39: "Not like that!" Effective propulsion looks different! Distinct trunk rotation—the sprinting player's arms move sideways (see the dotted line).

Table 11: Duration of running school instruction in the context of a training unit

Age	Duration per training unit in minutes
8-10	10
10-11	12-15
12-13	15-18
14-15	18-20

For the interested reader, exercises and drills for running school in soccer that can be directly integrated into soccer training.

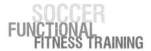
EXERCISE 1: RUNNING SCHOOL AS A TEAM

This format is very common in soccer training, and next to good visual movement control from the coach or instructor and, most important, the team, it leads to significant precision of movement, team spirit, and a willingness to put forth effort (pay attention to motivation).

VARIATION A: ONE LINE

- The players run one after the other in a line on a playing field with minimal distance inbetween (back and forth or in an oval). The last player starts and runs around the team on the outside all the way to the front and slows down to a fast walk. Now the next player does the same. Running can be varied usinghigh-knee running, butt kicking, Nordic walking, skipping, ankle-strengthening work, and running backwards and sideways.

VARIATION B: TWO LINES

- See variation A, whereby the players run in two lines side by side. This inevitably intensifies the exercise.

VARIATION C: ONE OR TWO LINES – VARYING SPEEDS

- The players run one after the other in one line. After a signal from the coach or instructor or the captain,the runner at the front takes a step to the side and slows down significantly (walking speed!). The team now runs past this player. The player then rejoins the line after the last runner has passed him. Then follow the next signal, and repeat.

VARIATION D:RUNNING IN TWO LINES WITH TEMPO CHANGES

- The players run side by side in two lines with a distance of approximately 6.5 feet between runners. At a signal from the coach or instructor or the captain, the last runner in each line sprints around the outside of his group to the front and then takes the lead at a slow jog. Repeat. (See photo 40.)

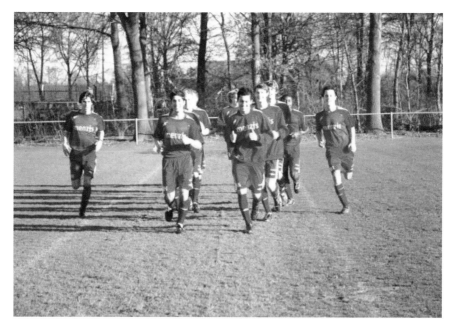

Photo 40: The two players at the back of the lines simultaneously sprint to the front.

VARIATION E: RUNNING IN TWO OFFSET LINES WITH TEMPO CHANGES

- See variation D, whereby the lines are offset (see photo 41). Line A (left side in photo 41) has now run almost completely past line B. When the last runner of line A is parallel to the first runner of line B, the entire line A slows down significantly, and the entire line B starts to sprint at the same time. The lines continuously push and shift past each other, and one player in each line is always "in charge." Communication and teamwork are a must here.

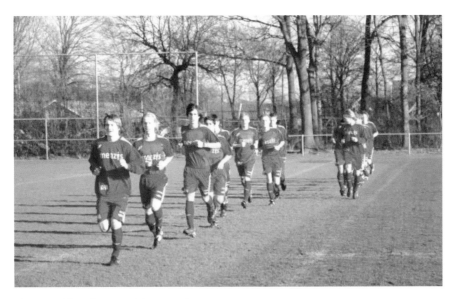

Photo 41: Offset lineruns with tempo changes.

VARIATION F: TWO LINES CIRCLING EACH OTHER AT A RUN

❯ See variation D, whereby, after a signal from the coach or instructor or captain, line A sprints around line B (photo 42). Once all players have returned to their original positions without colliding, line B can take off after a signal has been given.

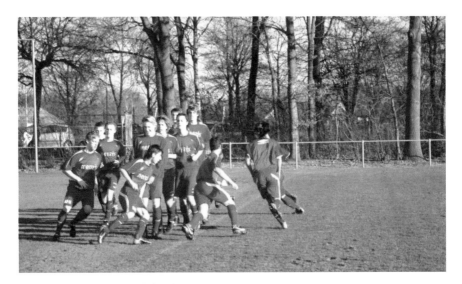

Photo 42: Sudden change of direction as a team.

EXERCISE 2: SLALOM RUN

Players run one in front of the other approximately 10 feet apart. At a signal from the coach or instructor or captain, the last player in the line sprints to the front in between the other runners in slalom form. The number of team members depends on the training goal.

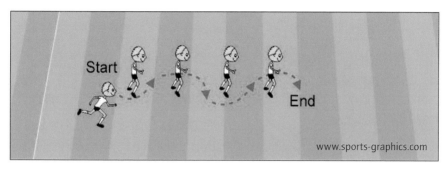

Fig. 22: Run fast without coming into contact with anyone!

EXERCISE 3: TAGGING AND RUNNING AWAY

Players walk side by side in two lines. One player from line A tags the player from line B walking next to him. Immediately after, both players try to run to the front of their line (around the outside of the lines). See who is the first to arrive at the front of his line. The coach or instructor specifies the number of sprints and the length of the series and breaks according to the training goal and makes sure that communication within and between lines is clear and intelligible.

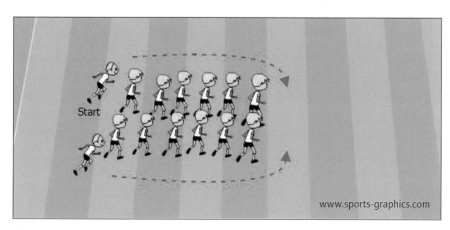

Fig. 23: Tagging and running away!

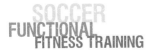

EXERCISE 4: TAGGING AND PURSUING

Players walk or run in one or two lines. Players should be about 10 feet apart. The last man in a line tags the player in front of him and runs past him. Both players move to the front of their team. Next the new last player of a line tagsthe player in front of him, and repeats. See who will make it to the front without getting tagged. The coach or instructor specifies the number of series and the length of the sprints and breaks according to the training goal and makes sure that communication within and between lines is clear and intelligible.

EXERCISE 5: SPRINTING AND TIMING

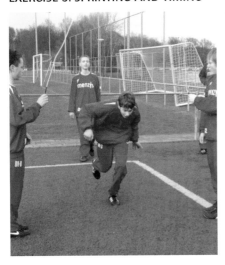

Photo 43: Complete the task without interruption!

The player receives a hard pass. He must settle the ball and carry it into the penalty box and then take a situational shot on goal.

In order for this highly complex task to succeed regularly and effectively, it is very important to develop preparatory and concomitant forms of training and drills in youth soccer training. The following form is a possible example:

The players constantly alternate running toward a swinging skipping rope from a distance of approximately 11 yards. They must run through the rope, which is swung counterclockwise by two teammates without interruption. The coach or instructor can turn this into a competition with rules: See who is able to make a pass without visibly stopping and without coming into contact with the rope.

VARIATIONS:

- Two players run one in front of the other toward the swinging rope.
- Relay competition with a baton: Two teams sprint back and forth.
- The distance to the rope is increased, making the task more difficult.
- Running through two ropes back to back. But the ropes must be an adequate distance apart.

EXERCISE 6: NUMBERS RUN

The team is divided into several groups, whereby each player is given a number between 1 and 4. By calling out a number, the coach or instructor indicates an action for specific players, and the action is then carried out.

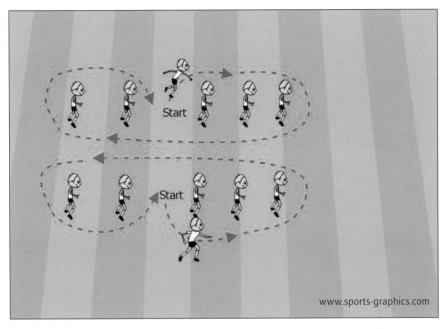

www.sports-graphics.com

Fig. 24: Concentration and running ability are needed here!

POSSIBLE TASKS:

- The players form two lines and stand in a row. Both groups walk in a specific direction. When the coach orinstructor calls out a certain number, those players run to the front (see fig. 24).
- Same as the previous task, but this time the players run around their own line and then resume their original position (see fig. 24). See who is first to return to his original spot.

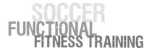

EXERCISE 7: NUMBERS RUN FROM A STANDING POSITION

Same as exercise 6 with the players starting from a standing position.

POSSIBLE TASK:

◈   Straight run, out and back with a turn.

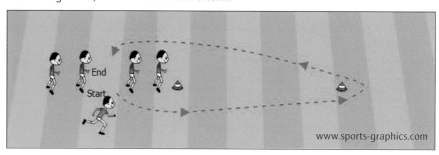

Fig. 25: Run out and back and exchange highfives!

The following figures are five examples of number runs with variable geometric shapes:

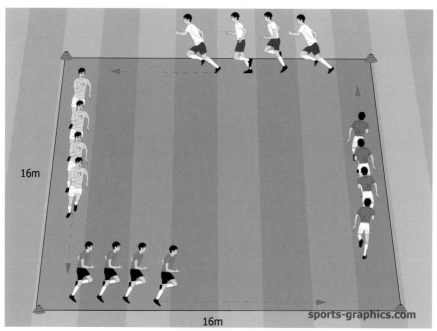

Fig. 26: Running in a square (16 x 16 m or 20 x 20 m)

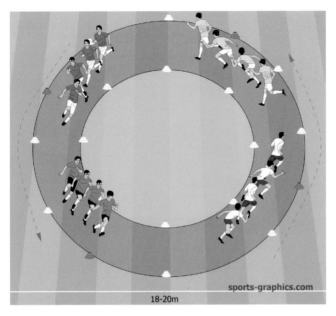

Fig. 27: Running in a circle (approximately 18-20m in diameter)

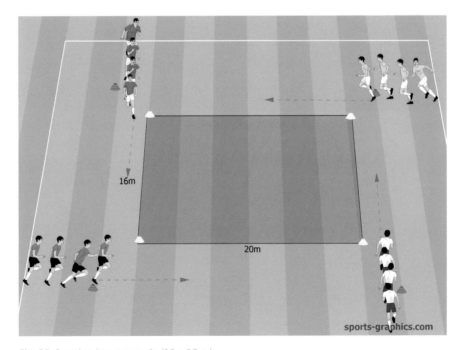

Fig. 28: Running in a rectangle (16 x 20 m)

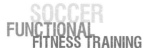

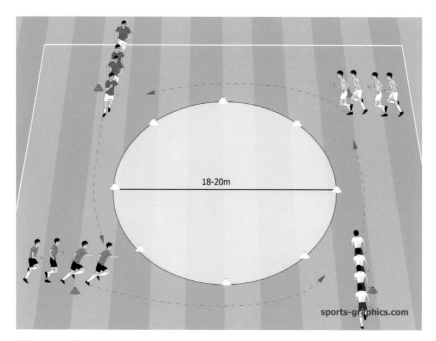

Fig. 29: Running a curve

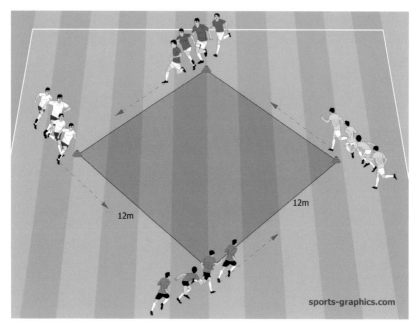

Fig. 30: Running in a diamond (edge length approximately 12 m)

EXERCISE 8: NUMBER RUNS THAT START WITH MOVEMENT

The runners run and the coach or instructor calls out a number.

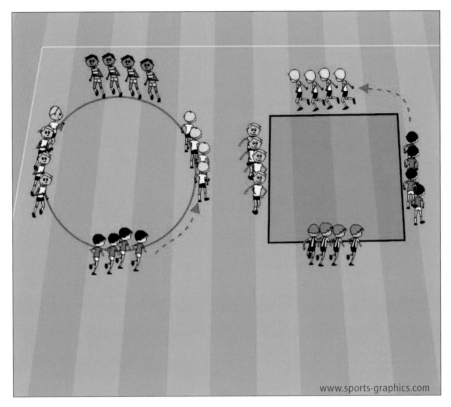

Fig. 31: From a movement into a sprint

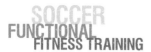
In all exercises and drills, the running direction should be changed constantly because

- ◐ one-sided loading of skeletal muscles should be avoided, and
- ◐ spatial awareness (moving left or right, forward and backward) must also be practiced in different ways.
- ◐ The players run in groups in a circle, clockwise or counterclockwise, and at a signal from the coach or instructor, run around a cone in the center of the circle and then run back to their group.
- ◐ The running distance depends on the training objective.

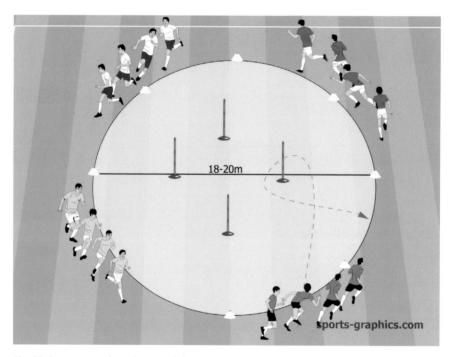

Fig. 32: Run, turn, and catch up again!

VARIATIONS:

- The players carry a baton or ball and hand it off to their group. The circle has an 18- to 20-meter diameter. See which group is the quickest.

- Same as previous, whereby players must now run up to the cones outside of the circle.

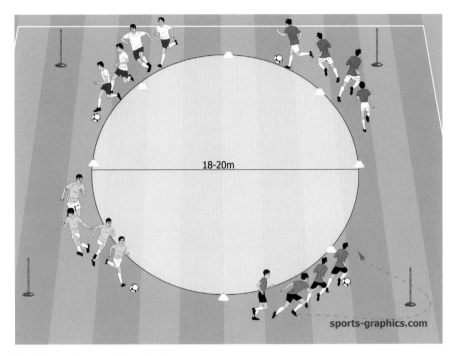

18-20m

sports-graphics.com

Fig. 33: Run to the outside and then rejoin your group.

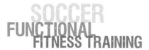

EXERCISE 9: TEAM RUN

The coach or instructor forms equal number teams. The teams run freely and one in front of the other on a marked field. At a signal from the coach or instructor, the second player of each team runs to the front, and at the same time the previously first runner goes to the back of the team. The other players close the gap left by the second player's moving up.

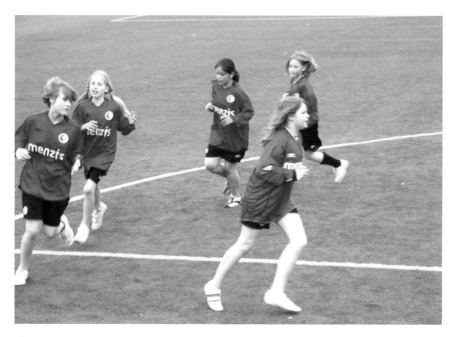

Photo 44: Always follow very closely behind the number one.

VARIATIONS:

❯ The team runs with high knees or skipping. The first player of a team specifies these movement variations, and all other players copy them precisely.

❯ Timed runs. The teams are given a task and perform it continuously for one minute, or any other specified time period. The coach or instructor whistles or claps when time is up. Then all players stop. See which player and which team can keep the shortest distances between each other.

OBJECTIVE:

❯ Stay together as a team and keep an eye on your teammate!

EXERCISE 10: SIX-DAY RACE – DEVELOPS A COMMON SENSE OF TEMPO IN A TEAM

Form two teams of equal size. The lineup resembles that of a six-day race: The teams stand facing each other on a marked off track (round, oval, triangular, square, hexagonal) in a slightly offset position. Once they have started, they will meet halfway. The coaches or instructors can ask for the following tasks to be accomplished:

- Adjust running speed to return to the starting position at the same time.
- Run for a predetermined period of time and focus on synchronized running.
- Ask players if they can "sense" the amount of time they have run (sense of tempo).
- Ask players if they can synchronize their running so there is no "too fast," "too slow," "too asynchronous," or "too heterogeneous."

EXERCISE 11: TIMEOUT

Form several teams that run together for approximately 4 to 8 minutes on a marked course on the soccer field. The course is designed so the teams must pass the coach or instructor. Players from the teams can ask the coach or instructor for a timeout (short break) as they run. If the coach or instructor agrees, the player can sit out one round and then rejoin the team. A player can ask for several timeouts.

See which player or group requires the fewest timeouts.

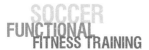

EXERCISE 12: ROAD TRAFFIC

Together, teams of four to six players run around the items (cones, mini goals, balls, benches) set up on the playing field. Players must constantly ascertain what their running positions are within the team (1,2, to 6). At a signal from the coach or instructor, the lead runner from each team constantly changes. For example, 1 switches with 4. Since several teams are running simultaneously, all teams must obey the right-of-way rules in traffic: right before left. Failure to observe these rules results in predetermined feedback from the coach or instructor. For example, 10 push-ups on the spot.

This exercise can also be completed in a field or a park.

The duration and number of runs and the break lengths depend on the respective training goal.

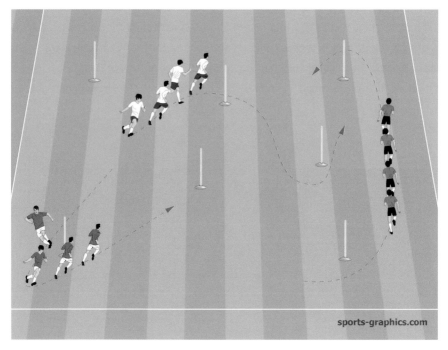

Fig. 34: Stay alert in road traffic.

EXERCISE 13: SPRINTERS TAKE PRIORITY

Form teams of four to six players and, depending on the training goal, set up a coursewith cones at the appropriate distances (see fig. 35). The first player of a team sprints from A to B and then calmly jogs back to the starting point in a slalom (see fig. 35). The second player takes off when the first player begins his jogging phase. To avoid dangerous collisions during the sprints, the rule is that sprinting players always have priority over jogging players. The coach or instructor determines the number of series and sprints, the distance, and the break lengths according to the training goal.

Distance between cones is 10 to 12 meters.

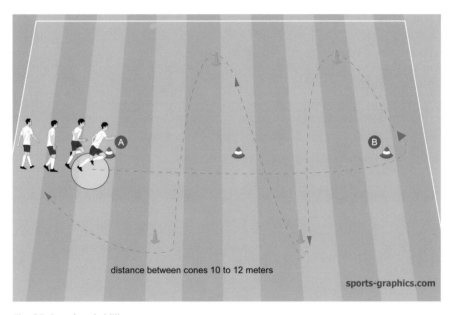

distance between cones 10 to 12 meters

sports-graphics.com

Fig. 35: Speed and chilling

EXERCISE 14: HUNT FOR POINTS

Four teams of four players each line up in rows behind a marked start and finish line. One player from each team runs around the cones, followed by the second, third, and fourth player. Each cone is worth a certain number of points (1 to 5 points; see fig. 36). The distance between the cones, the duration, and the number of series are determined by the coach or instructor.

- Short distances between cones: intensive interval training
- Longer distances between cones: extensive interval training

See which team earns the most points within specified time limit.

The coach or instructor should point out that the players courageously learn to experience their individual endurance ability and draw their conclusions with respect to future running school training:

- "I have to get faster!"
- "I have to learn to keep up!"

The results of this inner dialogue can become the basis for a future running school (learning to compete, communicate, and appraise).

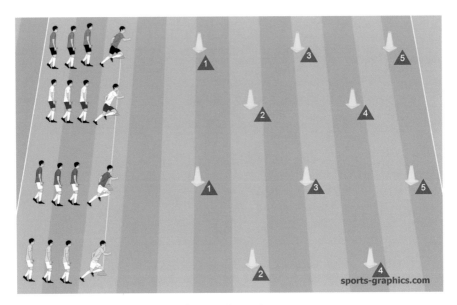

Fig. 36: Learning to compete, communicate, and appraise

EXERCISE 15: TRIANGLE RUNS

Divide players into teams. The teams run in triangles (see fig. 37). The triangles consist of AAA (26 x 26 x 26 m), BBB (24 x 24 x 24 m), and CCC (22 x 22 x 22 m). Each team starts at a corner. Players run the triangle at a specified tempo (e.g., 10 sec per side).

See which team can run at a tempo that allows them to run steadily without accelerating or slowing down at the corners of the triangle. Times, tempo, and break lengths depend on the training goals.

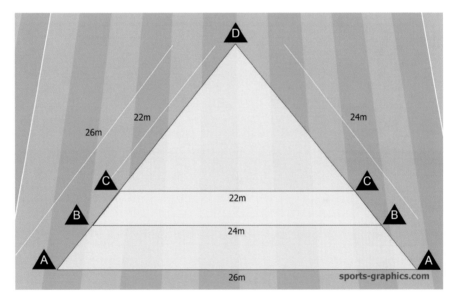

Fig. 37: Developing a sense of tempo!

VARIATIONS:

- ◉ Each player runs alone.
- ◉ Ask for pair runs.
- ◉ Individually, then as a pair, then in threes, and so on.
- ◉ Mark the geometric shape of the square.
- ◉ As a relay with a specified tempo.

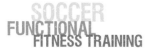

EXERCISE 16: SQUARE RUNS

Use cones to mark three overlapping squares. The sides should be approx. 10, 15, and 20 meters (see fig. 38). This creates three laps (small, medium, and large). Then form four teams with four players each. The number one (to be determined) of each team starts and leads the team. After three rounds, the number two takes the lead, and so on. The coach or instructor signals the number of laps the teams must run.

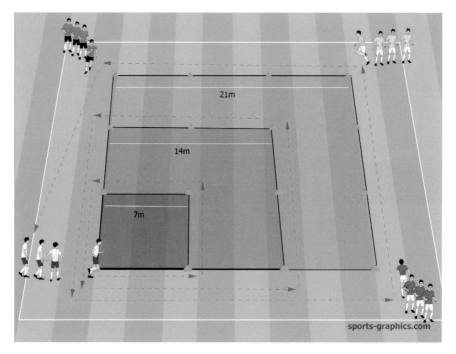

Fig. 38: Alternating the lead

VARIATIONS:

- Deliberately change the tempo: one side fast, the other side slow.
- Change direction: Run clockwise and counterclockwise.
- See which player or team is best able to estimate the amount of time needed to run three laps.
- Run 3 x 3 laps in a specified amount of time. See which team meets the time allotment or gets closest to doing so.

EXERCISE 17: PARTNER RUNS WITH TIMEOUTS

Mark a 50- to 100-metercourse and form teams of three players. Two from each team run the course with time allotments: run 6, 8, 10, or 12 minutes without stopping. The coach or instructor determines the time allotted based on the team's training level and goal. The third player from each team, who is waiting at the edge of the course, can relieve the other two players. See which team will stay closest within the time allotment and runs the farthest.

EXERCISE 18: GROUPS OF THREERUNS WITH TIMEOUTS

See exercise 17, whereby the teams are comprised of four to five players who must continually run together. The coach or instructor should see to it that the teams run at and maintain a fast pace.

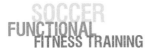
EXERCISE 19: LET SOMEONE ELSE DO THE RUNNING –HAVE SOME FUN!

Mark different routes on a playing field: line, circle, triangle, square, double-circles for figure-eights. Form teams (e.g., with four players) and give the first player a die. The player throws a number that the players behind him must run in laps. Next, the second player throws the die, and so on. Every player gets a turn.

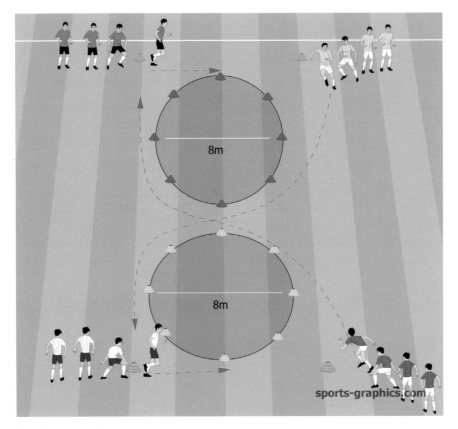

Fig. 39: Figure-eights

The diameter of a circle is approximately 8 meters.

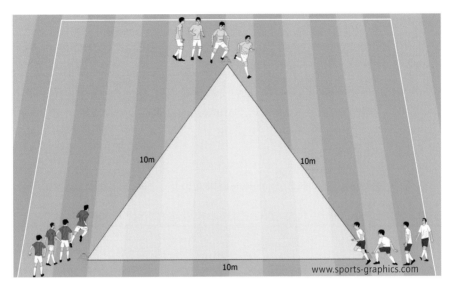

Fig. 40: Triangle runs

The length of one side is approximately 10 meters.

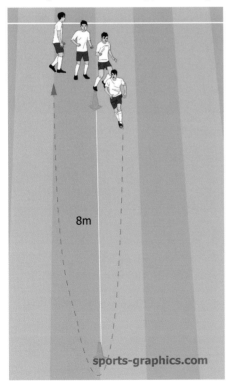

Fig. 41: Line runs

The distance between the two cones is approximately 8 meters.

VARIATION:

❯ Teams throw the die for each other.

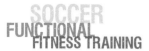

EXERCISE 20: TAXI

Mark the following routes one to three and form teams of four to six players. Each team's number one runs a specific route. When he gets back to his starting point, the next passenger gets in the taxi, meaning, the waitingplayers gradually attach themselves to the back of the line of playersrunning past. The coach or instructor determines the distance between the cones and benches, and the number of series based on the training goal.

See which team is the first to completely return to the starting point.

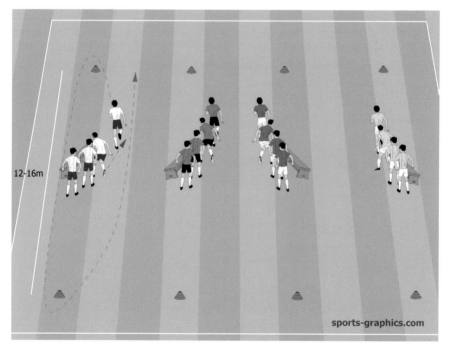

Fig. 42: Route 1

The distance between the cones is approximately 12 to 16 meters.

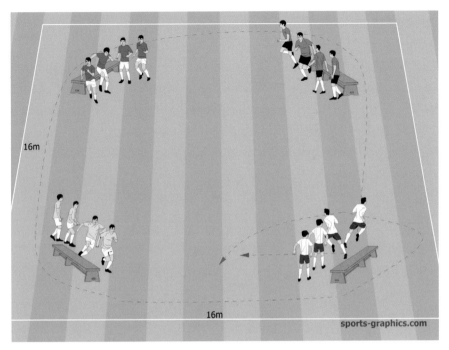

Fig. 43: Route 2

The benches are in the corners of the field. The field is approximately 16 x 16 meters.

VARIATION:

◉ On route 2 (fig. 43), the front runner always runs around the bench and after connecting with the next player, changes his running direction. This variation requires more concentration since all players should run at the same tempo. Tell players to take a look around so they can adapt their tempo to that of the other players.

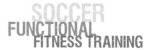

EXERCISE 21: RUNNING FIGURE-EIGHTS

Mark the pictured geometric shape (see fig. 44) and form four teams of four players each. The first players of team A (red) and B (blue) lead their teams and start to run simultaneously (see fig. 44). When, for instance, team A reaches team C (green), the first player from that team joins team A at the rear. This new team then runs toward team D (white), where the first player of that team again joins up at the rear. The frontrunner always makes sure that the distance to the other teams remains the same. When both teams are complete, they run one more lap. After that, one player from each team always falls away after each figure-eight so that only the original A and B tams remain at the end. Teamwork is necessary.

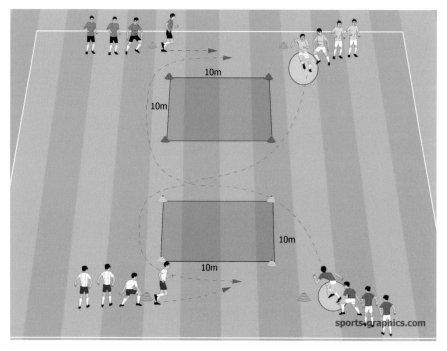

Fig. 44: Teamwork

The sides of the squares are approximately 10 meters.

EXERCISE 22: STAR RUN

The coaches or instructors mark a star shape and form four teams of equal size (see fig. 45). The size of the star and the number of repetitions and series are chosen based on the training goal, whereby the rules of the game can be implemented in pairs, teams, or collectively (see forms 19 and 20 in chapter 9).

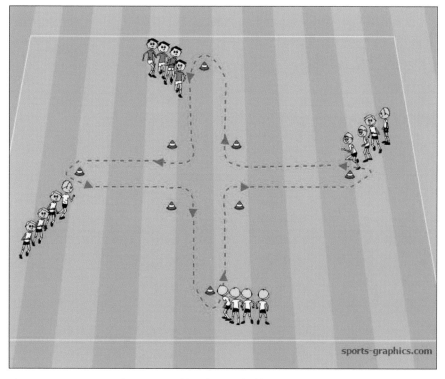

Fig. 45: Tempo run past the cones marking the star, inside and outside

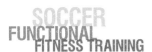

EXERCISE 23: SYNCHRONIZED RUNS

The coach or instructor marks approximately four rows of cones as shown in fig. 46 and forms two teams of approximately three players each (run-to-rest ratio is 1:2). The distances between the cones and from the cones to the players and the number of repetitions and series depend on the training goal. The two front players of both teams start at the same time and run the course in a zigzag line (see fig. 46). The player on the right always has the rightofway. The second pair of players starts when the first pair has reached the second row of cones. After reaching the end of the last row of cones, the pair runs along the cones on the outside and back to the finish line.

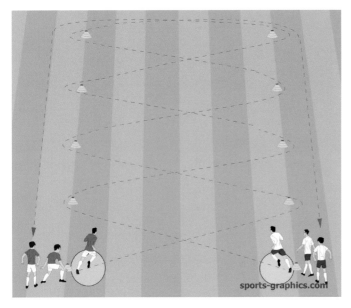

Fig. 46: Learning cooperation and sense of tempo

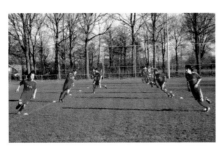

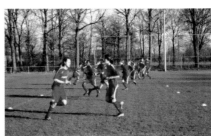

Photo 45: Synchronized running   *Photo 46: Meet in the middle!*

EXERCISE 24: INTERVAL PARTNER RUNS

The coaches or instructors mark a 15- to 30-meter square (ABCD; see fig. 47) and form two teams of equal size.

The first players of each group run synchronized on lines ABC (red) and ADC (white) and back to their starting cone. Then the next pair runs. The number of players, repetitions, and series depend on the training goal. In fig. 47, only one cone has been marked with C and with A. The unmarked cones should be evenly assigned to C and A.

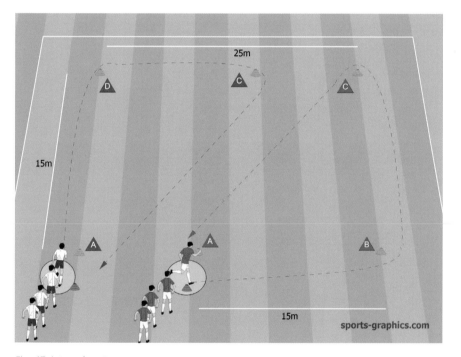

Fig. 47: Interval partner runs

VARIATIONS:

- Both players complete the diagonal at the end in a full-out sprint.
- The pair runs ins-and-outs (step-down fartlek).

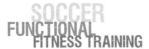
EXERCISE 25: INSIDE–OUTSIDE LANE

Mark a large circle (or two large circles that can be run as figure-eights).

Players run alone or with a partner (side by side). Running in a circle or in a figure-eight will teach the players what it means to run on the inside or the outside (inside and outside lane). They will also encounter this phenomenon in a competitive game, with respect to the opponent and the ball: difference in tempo, the planting of the foot, the stride, and the shifting center of gravity. They, therefore, constantly alternate between the inside and outside lane, independently or prompted by the coach or instructor. The size of the circle and the number of players, repetitions, and series depend of the training goal.

EXERCISE 26: RUNNING LAPS

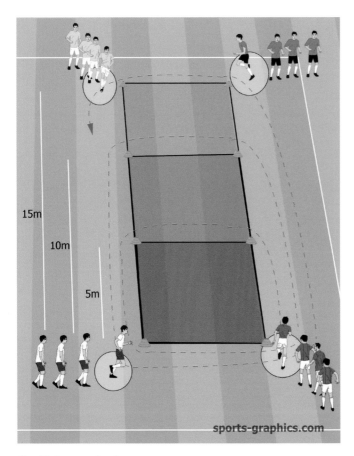

Fig. 48: Run your laps!

Use eight or more cones to mark the depicted shape (see fig. 48) and form four teams. Players on each team run alone, in pairs, or as a group within a time interval determined by the coach or instructor (or a specific number of laps). Distances between cones (e.g., 5-10-15 m), the number of players per team, repetitions, and series depend on the training goal.

VARIATION:

◐ Jog the longer distances and run the shorter ones.

EXERCISE 27: INTERMEDIATE SPRINT

Form four teams of four players each and number them one through four. The four teams run one behind the other, 15 to 20 meters apart, around a large circle, large square, or large rectangle. At a signal from the coach or instructor or the team captain, the first player of each team (number one) sprints to the rear of the team in front of his and joins that team.

VARIATION:

◐ The coach or instructor does not only signal the number but also the sprint to the team ahead of the next team. This extends the running distance and increases the attentiveness of the players.

EXERCISE 28: RELAY

On a marked round track with a 15- to 40-meter diameter, players of four teams (see form 27, chapter 9) run one behind the other at a moderate tempo. The number one players carry a baton or a ball and at a signal from the coach or instructor, sprint around the outside of the track and hand the baton or ball off to the number three player, and so on. The coach or instructor can turn this into a continuous relay sprint competition.

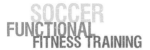

EXERCISE 29: RUNNING IN A DIAMOND 1

Mark a diamond shape. Distances between cones are 15 to 20 meters. Form four teams of equal size and position them as shown in fig. 49.

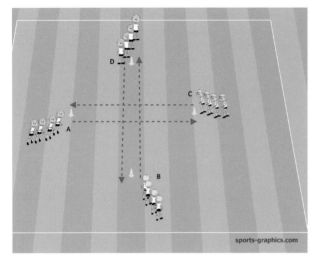

After a signal from the coach or instructor, the front (number one) players of teams A and C start by switching places at a sprint (see fig. 49). The front players of teams B and D start to run when the players from A and C reach the center of the diamond, and so on.

Fig. 49: Team sprints in a diamond.

VARIATION:

See exercise 20, whereby each player will take the forward position on his team one time during the team round robin.

EXERCISE 30: RUNNING IN A DIAMOND 2

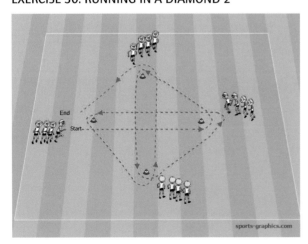

See exercise 29, whereby the teams' running course looks as shown in fig. 50. First run diagonally, then turn left and run diagonally again. Each player does this four times and then finishes at his respective starting point.

Fig. 50: Specified course for diagonal runs (the diamond measures approximately 12 x 12 m)

VARIATIONS:

- Run counterclockwise.
- Sprint the diagonals and jog the outsides.
- All teams alternate sprinting and jogging.
- In "taxi" form (see exercise 20) with a steady tempo.
- Same taxi formbut sprint the diagonals.
- If the distances between the cones are greater than 16 meters, the two teams facing each other are able to begin at the same time. If the two teams are on the other side, the two other teams facing each other start.

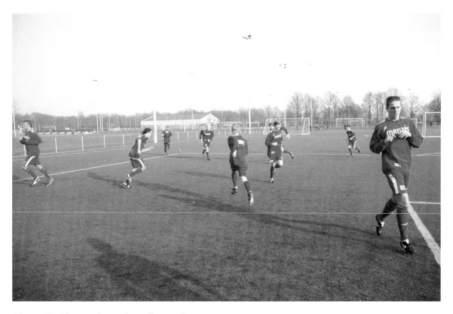

Photo 47: Diagonal runs in a diamond

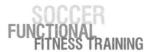
EXERCISE 31: AGILITY LADDER

Lay out agility ladders. These generally consist of 12 rungs (speed ladder, with closely spaced rungs) or 24 rungs with even or uneven spacing. These can be positioned in a variety of ways, depending on team size, fitness level, and objectives.

At first players should try to discover the space between rungs individually using small steps and step combinations and even and varying stride frequencies. After running through the ladder, the players should adopt a stride frequency and rhythm that will be followed by a 10- to 15-meter sprint.

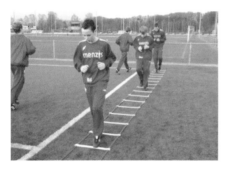

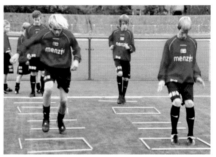

Photo 48: Agility ladder and varying stride frequencies

Photo 49: Stride frequency training using poles combined with skipping and running jumps (forward and sideways)

VARIATION:

- The already familiar running ABCs can be implemented here using agility ladders, poles, cones, and mini hurdles.

CAUTION!

When implementing the drills from exercise 31, it is especially advisable to always change the distances between the methodological tools and greatly vary the rhythms. Otherwise, in the authors' experience, there is no productive progression in terms of an increased stride frequency.

EXERCISE 32: SKIPPING OVER MINI HURDLES

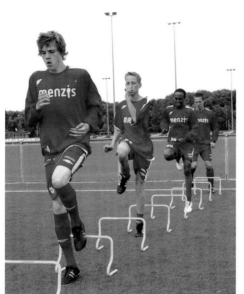

Set up 6 to 12 mini hurdles (variable height) in a row (see photo 50) and ask the players to run the mini hurdles as if they were not there. The coach or instructor should emphasize high-knee lifts and hands raised to chin level (see photo 50). This exercise can be combined with different running rhythms between the hurdles: 1-2-3-4-5. The mini hurdles must then be positioned farther apart to facilitate a steady movement sequence.

Photo 50: Skipping over hurdles

The coach or instructor should also look for the following movement characteristics:

- Head position
- Shoulder position
- Arm position
- Trunk posture
- Knee movement
- Foot placement
- Perceptible relaxed demeanor

The number of hurdles and their height, the distances between the mini hurdles, the number of repetitions and series, and the break lengths depend on the training goal.

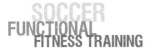
EXERCISE 33: DIFFERENTIATED SPRINTS

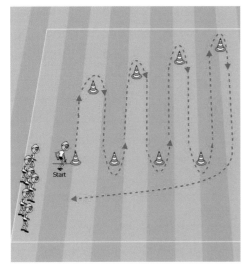

Set up cones at distances of 10, 12, 14, and 16 meters (see fig. 51). The coach or instructor determines the number of repetitions and series and the breaks based on the training goal and team size. The first player of a team starts at A and tries to run each stretch after a turning point faster than the previous one. After completion of the course, the player jogs back to his team.

Fig. 51: Steadily increase your running tempo!

VARIATIONS:

- ◉ Guideline: Players assess themselves and get to know their sprinting abilities.
- ◉ Players must spread out independently behind cones A, B, C, or D. At a signal from the coach or instructor, they run the course all the way through and try to pass the player in the adjacent lane (e.g., C next to B) or try not to let the distance between them increase. See who is able to complete this task.Different competition rules with reward systems can be used here.For example,create a spreadsheet on which the weekly winner(s) of the day can be entered. Post this in the locker room and keep it updated. The macro- and mesocycle winner gets a prize.
- ◉ Hold a relay race with teams of equal size. Four teams position at cones A to D, each with a ball or baton. For example, the first player from team D runs toward A, then runs around the outside of the cone and back to the back of his team where he hands off the baton or ball to the next runner. The coach or instructor must make sure that players are lined up in such a way that players are able to safely run around the teams and return to their starting point and switch (add additional markings if necessary). After a heat is completed, the teams move up (e.g., B to C, or D to A). Reward systems can be used here a well.

EXERCISE 34: CHASE THE HOOP

The team is divided into pairs. Each pair has a gymnastics hoop. One player from each pair rolls the hoop as far as possible down the field. The teammate must try to run after the hoop and catch it before it falls flat on the ground. See which pair rolls and runs farthest. The number of repetitions, series, and breaks depend on the training goal.

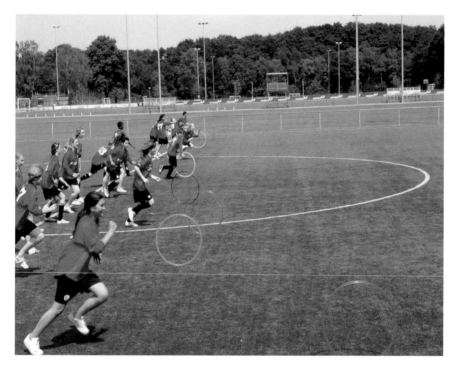

Photo 51: Chase the hoop – teamwork, technique, and running ability rule!

VARIATIONS:

- Mark a 20-meter distance. The action is the same as the main exercise, but seewhich pair is able to return to the starting point quickest with the hoop. The hoop can only be rolled.
- Same as main exercise, but in relay form.

CHAPTER

13

13 JUMPING GAMES FOR SOCCER PLAYERS

> *"Sufficient stimulus strength in training, e.g. via body weight exercises, or even small jumps, is thus appropriate (in youth training)."*

(Ollmanns, 2009b, p. 9)

In chapter 9, the authors introduce jumping and leaping elements taken from different game sports. The following exercises and training forms in this chapter link chapters 9 and 14. Together, both chapters form the real basis for the soccer-specific types of jumps in chapter 14.

EXERCISE1: JUMP ROPE

Today jumping rope has largely been replaced by **rope skipping** (and leather rope). Both types of ropes are suitable for youth training, whereby it must be emphasized that the wrist and forearm work with the rope presents a greater technical challenge for young athletes.

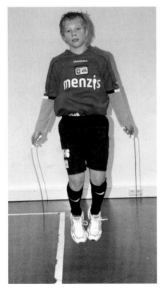

Photo 52: Jumping rope with the rope skipper. This must include working on technique and movement efficiency.

Rope jumping variations are diverse and most often include skills like single- anddouble-leg jumping, running, high-knee lifts at varying heights, skipping, gaining space while jumping (right-left, forward-back; with turns), and running jumps. Combined with crossing the arms, a partner (one in front of the other), rhythmic and arrhythmic sequences, different jumping heights and distances, and creative combinations of different skills,these make interesting projects for youth players that can be doneas homework, counting the number of jumps

177

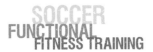

or joined movements, degree of difficulty (perfect movement combinations), and precision (faultless vs. faulty). They can be performed during practice as an internal show-and-tell in front of the team and coach or instructor. Competitions with ranking lists and awards can be used here, too.

EXERCISE 2: JUMPING CIRCLE

The team forms a circle. One player or the coach or instructor swings a rope with a small bag filled with seeds, or something similar, attached to the other end to add weight while spinning in place. Players jump (two legs, one leg) when the rope reaches their feet.

VARIATIONS:

- Tuck jump
- Jump turns
- Jump holding hands

The number of jumps depends on the training goal.

EXERCISE 3: TEAM JUMPING

On a marked field, set up approximately six long benches (or rows of cones with horizontal posts or rows of mini hurdles) 2.5 to 3 meters apart. Players jump over the obstacles together in teams of two, three, or four (hands clasped) in a particular running rhythm. The number of joint jumps depends on the training goal.

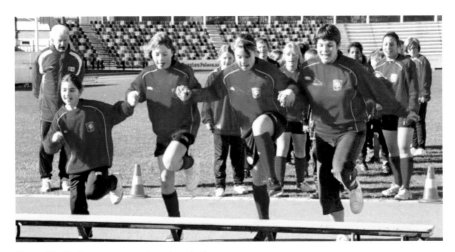

Photo 53: Finding a common jumping rhythm as a team.

EXERCISE 4: JUMPING AT THE RIGHT MOMENT

Same as exercise 3, whereby a cone and a teammate (catcher) are positioned on each bench.Each player must now try to jump over as many benches as possible without being tagged by the catcher. They have 30 seconds to do so. If the catcher tags a player,his jump does not count.

The players are not allowed to jump over the same bench twice in a row. See which player can complete the most jumps.

The coach or instructor determines the duration based on the training goal.

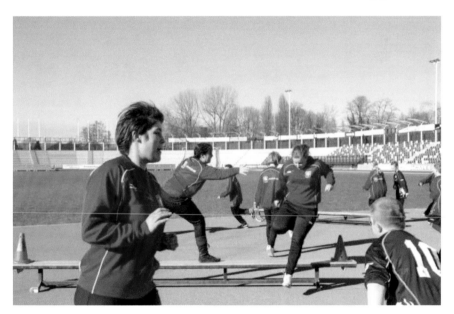

Photo 54: Who can avoid the catcher on the bench?

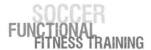
EXERCISE 5: SPEED JUMPING

The coach or instructor specifies a number of mini hurdles (varying heights) to be set up on a marked field. Depending on the training goal, the coach or instructor now asks the team to jump as many hurdles as possible in 20 seconds. The players are not allowed to jump the same hurdle twice in a row.

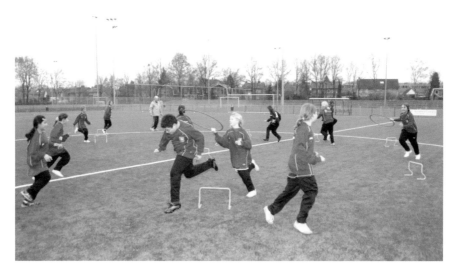

Photo 55: Jumps over mini hurdles

VARIATION:

❯ Same as main exercise, whereby the coach or instructor specifies a number of catchers who will try to catch the jumping players with gymnastics hoops. If they succeed, only the number of mini hurdles jumped before a player was caught is counted. Then that player starts to compete again or he switches with the catcher. See which player has the longest run per specified time unit (e.g., 45 seconds).

EXERCISE 6: ALTERNATING LEAPFROG

Form teams of four players and assign them a number, and then mark a field. All players initially run freely on the field. When the coach or instructor or captain calls out, for instance, "number one," all players with the number one get in a crouch, and the other players leapfrog over them. All numbers will get a chance to leap in the course of the game. In addition, the coach or instructor sets a time limit within which the players must complete their respective leaps. See which player completes the most (added up) frog leaps.

EXERCISE 7: HOOP JUMPING

Form teams of five players and assign each team a number from one to five. Teams line up in a row from one to five. The game starts with the first player from a team (number one) holding a hoop and at a signal from the coach or instructor, standing it upright and attempting to hurdle it with a straddle-jump. If he succeeds, the number two player takes the hoop and attempts the same task, and so on.

When the hoop has reached the fifth player, he takes the hoop and runs with it to the front of his team and completes the described sequence from the beginning. Hoop jumping ends when the number one player is back at the front of his team with the hoop. The coach or instructor should visibly mark the distance between the first and last player of a team. He could possibly time the first- and second-place finishers with a stopwatch. This can prevent controversy. He should also make sure that the straddle-jump is performed correctly (accepting rules).

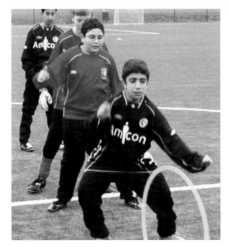

The number of heats depends on the training goal. Occasionally use different size hoops.

See which team posts the fastest heat.

Photo 56: Preparing for the straddle-jump over the vertically positioned and rolling hoop

EXERCISE 8: THE SINGLE-LEG ONES

Form four groups of four who will stand around a square marked with four cones (see photo 57). The players link hands and try to stand on one leg without losing their balance and without touching a cone with a foot. If a player puts down his second foot, falls down, or touches one of the cones with one of his legs, he gets a penalty point, and the game is briefly interrupted. Players switch their hopping leg after each interruption. The coach's assessment of the number of repetitions and series and the break lengths should be teamoriented based on the fitness level.See which player gets the fewest penalty points.

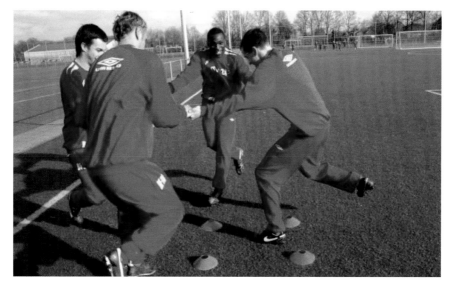

Photo 57: Hopping circle

VARIATION:

➙   Players get a penalty point if they step into the square with one foot or touch one of the cones. This generally results in more vigorous arm activity.

EXERCISES 9 AND 10: PUSHING AND PULLING DUELS

Form pairs that face each other in a marked corridor. In the first variation (photo 58), the players have their hands on the partner's shoulders. Players try to move each other off balance using single-leg hops, so a player has to leave the marked corridor (evasive maneuver) or has to use his second leg. In both cases, the player gets a penalty point. Make sure to regularly alternate the jumping leg.

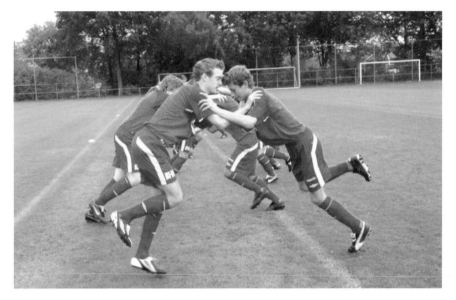

Photo 58: Push the partner across the line at a hop!

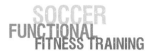

In the second variation (photo 59), both players firmly hold on to the partner's forearms and at a signal from the coach or instructor, try to pull the partner across the own line. Each successful attempt earns a bonus point. See who on the team gets the most bonus points in a "dog eat dog" scenario.

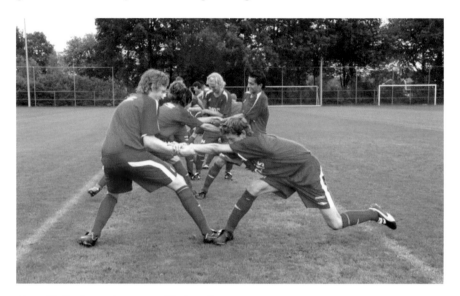

Photo 59: Forcing one's partner off balance!

Due to the high intensitythe coach's or instructor's determination of loading and unloading phases should be teamoriented.

VARIATION:
- ❯ Pull the partner hopping across your own line.
- ❯ Try to push your partner across the line using your shoulders with your arms crossed behind your back. Caution: Discuss head butts and avoid them at all cost.

EXERCISE 11: QUICK FEET

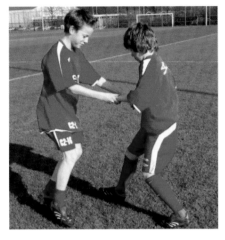

Partners firmly link hands, hop on one leg, and with their other foot, try to touch the partner's jumping foot (don't kick or stomp; see photo 60). After each touch, which scores a bonus point, switch the jumping foot.See who scores the most touches.

The coach or instructor must factor in and determine the number of repetitions and series and the break lengths beforehand.

Photo 60: Learning anticipatory behavior control

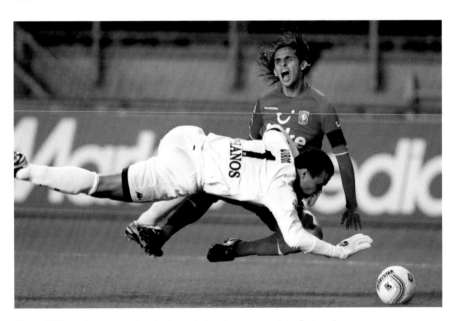

Photo 61: Learning to avoid pain throughsituation-appropriate footwork

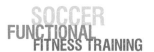

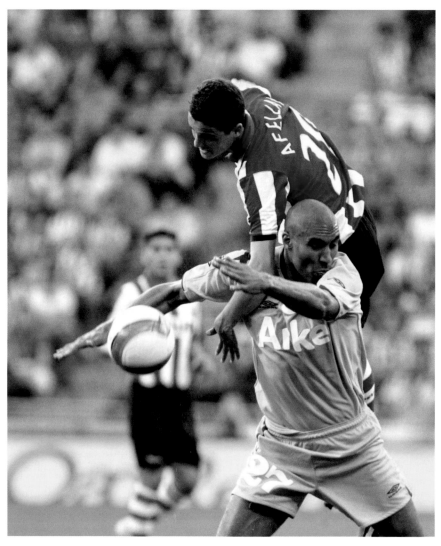

Photo 62: Air duels require courage, timing, technique, and explosive power. Players need to prepare with training.

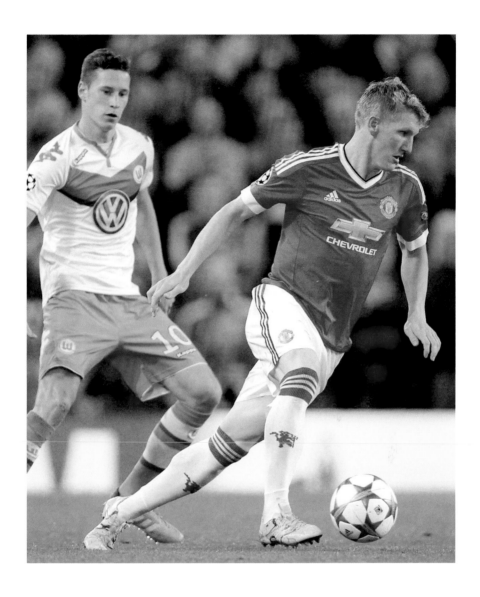

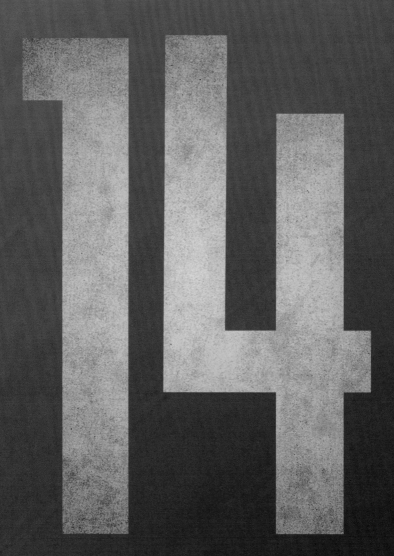

> CHAPTER

14

14 JUMPING EXERCISES FOR SOCCER PLAYERS

More than two-thirds of injuries and damages from overloading in soccer are to the lower extremities (Schmitt, 2013, p. 18). Since peak forces on the locomotor system of up to eight timestheir bodyweight can already occur in jumps of children andadolescents in everyday life (Fuchs et al., 2001) and apophyseal avulsions and injuries to the epiphyseal plates, in particular, must be avoided at all cost, it is fundamentally important that coaches or instructors exclude uncontrolled and non-physiological jumping techniques from accurate technique training (including breaks from physical loading).

When jumping exercises are preceded by *jumping games*, like in chapter 13, the coach or instructor creates an adequate foundation for increasing load intensities (prevention and increased load tolerance). Moreover, when following the research findings of Sadres et al. (2001),we can underscore here that no increased injury risk and negative effects on biological maturing processes can be detected, particularly when using a variety of age-specific strength elements and when working safely and precisely with pre-teen and adolescent youth players.

Since soccer is a game sport with lots of physical contact, it is important to note, as per Schmitt (2013, p. 18), that children and adolescents sustain bone injuries more often than adults. These tend to affect the upper extremities approximately three times more often than the lower. Furthermore, soccer players tend to exhibit position-specific injury patterns:

- Goal players: upper extremities and posterior cruciate ligament injuries
- Field players: mostly lower extremity injuries; defenders tend to have the most injuries

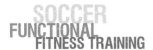
The coach or instructor must take it very seriously when youth players experience pain during jumping (strength) exercises over an extended period of time, particularly during a growth stage. Professional medial treatment is always a good idea. But often specific, moderate, eccentric strength training and coordination exercises can result in pain symptoms disappearing (accompanying preventative measures).

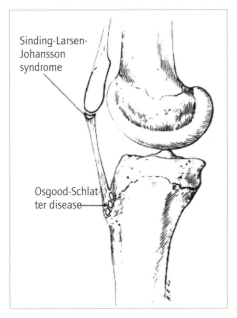

Sinding-Larsen-Johansson syndrome

Osgood-Schlatter disease

At this time, we would like to offer two examples that, in the author's estimation, often occur during the growth stages of youth players: knee pain and ankle pain.

As to knee pain: When youth players present with pain at the junction of the patellar tendon and the tibia, we often see swelling at that location.

Fig. 52: Two typical disorders of the knee joint in youth soccer players

It is problematic that the tibia's growth core is located precisely in that spot.

This disorder, which a coach or instructor should not discount, is called *Osgood-Schlatter* disease(see fig. 52).

If a youth player frequently complains about pain directly below the patella (see fig. 52), it can point to a disorder called Sinding-Larsen-Johansson syndrome. In both cases a medical diagnosis by a specialist is advisable.

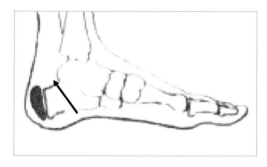

As to ankle pain: Players report pain in the area where the Achilles tendon attaches to the heel bone (see fig. 53). There is a growth core in this location as well. In the medical field, this disorder is referred to as *Sever's disease.*

Fig. 53: Another typical disorder in youth players: Sever's disease in the heel area

In addition, thereis often a hardening of the extensor muscles, flexor strains, and fiber tears, overstretching or strains of the Achilles tendon, strains of the plantar tendon in the arch of the foot, periosteal complaints, back problems, and ankle and ligament injuries. What can a coach or instructor do when these symptoms occur? As a preventative measure, it is possible to analyze in advance whether or not youth players are, in fact, in a major growth stage. Regular measuring and weighing, should, therefore, be an important part of an ambitious youth training program. Jumping exercises should be adapted accordingly with respect to volume, intensity, and surface.

It is often advisable to hold jumping exercises on a natural grass surface and to make sure that materials used in the construction of a new playing surface and running track have a cushioning effect. During winter training in the gym,it is important to make sure that gym mats (rolls), judo mats, or a sprung floor are available for jumping exercises. In this context, footwear must also be geared to the floor surface, foot posture (e.g., contracted foot, splayfoot, or talipes valgus), and possibly orthopedic inserts.

Furthermore, taking temporary breaks without jumps, constantly alternating between jumping exercises and coordination training, and consulting a medical specialist or physical therapist is also recommended.

Prevalent training (Schlumberger, 2006, p. 128-129; Killing, 2008, p. 172) for takeoff (jumping) during season prep (weeks 1-10/12) for advanced athletes in adult game sports

- begins with uphill jumps and strength circuits with emphasis on legs,
- is followed by series of jumps on grass, specific leg strength exercise, and
- finally, is a series of jumps on artificial surfaces that focus on distance and integrated maximum strength training.

The following exercises can be divided into four categories:

- First category: Jumping exercises without aids and into open space
- Second category: Jumping exercises with gymnastics hoops
- Third category: Jumping exercises with ropes and poles
- Fourth category: Jumping exercises with mini hurdles

14.1 JUMPING EXERCISES WITHOUT AIDS INTO OPEN SPACE

Basic forms: Players perform jumping exercises that include single-leg jumps (hopping jumps), double-leg jumps (forward, side to side, backward), running jumps, alternating jumps, tuck jumps, straddle-jumps, straddle-tuck jumps, and full-turn jumps (clockwise and counterclockwise).

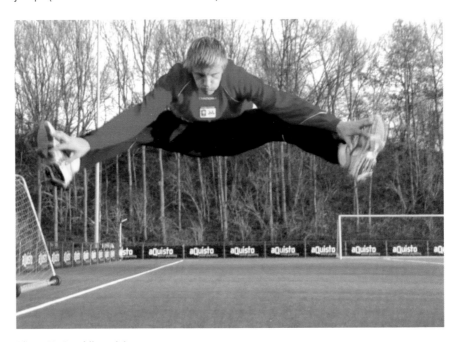

Photo 63: Straddle-tuck jump

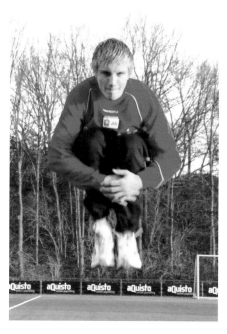

Photo 64: Tuck jump into open space

Variations: Jumping combinations have proven beneficial in training. These are usually very demanding with respect to coordination. At practice, the coach or instructor should, therefore, pay particular attention to technical execution and, depending on the training goal, break periods (rule of thumb: quality over quantity!). The following are possible jumping combinations:

- 2 x left and 2 x right single-legged jumps
- 3 x left and 3 x right single-legged jumps
- 4 hops, 4 x left single-legged jumps, 4 x right single-legged jumps, followed by 4 running jumps
- 2 x left single-legged jumps combined with 1 high double-leg jump
- 2 x right single-legged jumps combined with 1 double-leg jump
- 4 straddle jumps in all directions
- 4 tuck jumps in all directions
- 4 straddle-tuck jumps in all directions

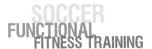

14.2 JUMPING EXERCISES WITH GYMNASTICS HOOPS

In the authors' opinion, situations that require jumping combinations are particularly well suited for developing a soccer player's power in practice. When they are used in different ways during training, it noticeably raises the motivational character and helps to determine the leading training stimuli in the best possible way. Here, too, individual and team-specific training directed by the coach or instructor is important. The Xs in the illustration represent the participating players, the circles represent the hoops, and the triangles show the cone markers.

EXERCISE1: PERFORM SINGLE-LEG AND DOUBLE-LEG JUMPS ON A TRACK

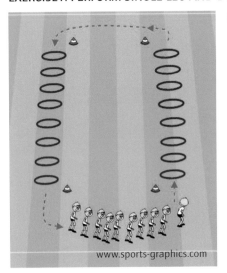

Fig. 54: Single-leg jumps around a track

www.sports-graphics.com

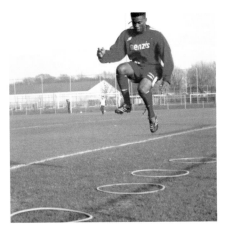

Photo 65: Coordinating height and distance of single-leg jumps

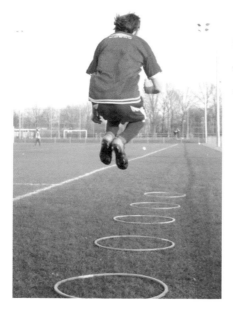

Photo 66: Double-leg jumps with the goal of gaining space

VARIATION:

⊘ Diagonal sequence with single-leg and double-leg jumps and two teams. This variation makes it easy to control muscle loading and unloading phases. The number of hoops and the distances between them depend on the training goal.

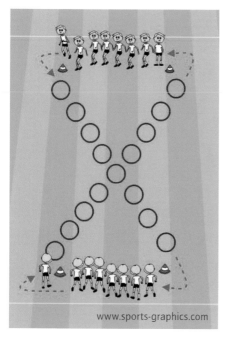

Fig. 55: Single-leg and Double-leg jumps on a diagonal

www.sports-graphics.com

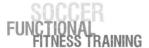
EXERCISE 2: SKATING JUMPS

See first form. This form combined with ice-skating is becoming increasingly popular in international high-performance soccer centers because it initiates particular locomotor muscle action that is very similar to directional changes in soccer.

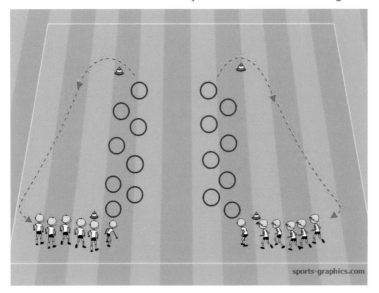

Fig. 56: Organized skating jumps

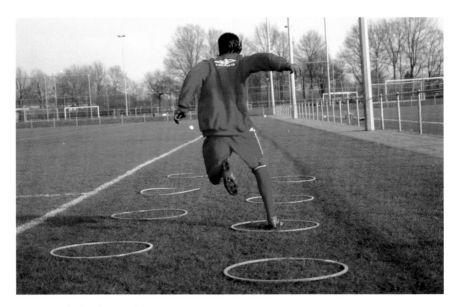

Photo 67: Skating jumps with arm support

EXERCISE 3: SEVEN JUMPS

See exercise 2. Starting at the first hoop, players must reach the six hoops with no more than seven running jumps. See who is able to reach even the farthest hoop with seven running jumps (increasing distance)? Adjust the distances of the hoops according to the team's jumping ability.

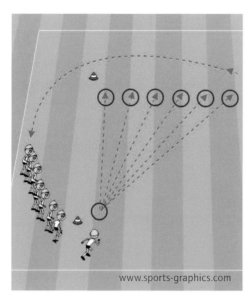

Fig. 57: Organized running jumps for distance

EXERCISE 4: COMBINATION JUMPS

See exercise 3. Players perform single-legcombination jumps, alternating legs. Distances between hoops depend on the group's jumping ability but should not be less than 2 to 2.5 meters.

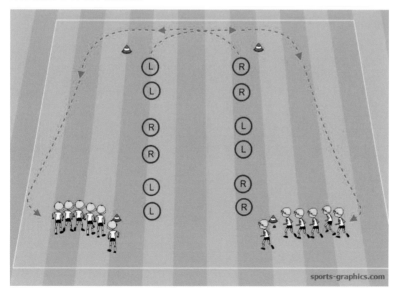

Fig. 58: Alternating single-leg combination jumps

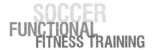
14.3 JUMPING EXERCISES WITH ROPES AND POLES

Each soccer player should own a jump rope. It can be used to promote soccer fitness on and off the soccer field in a variety of ways: hopping, running, single-leg jumps (also combinations), running jumps, short alternating jumps, and skipping. By coordinating arm and leg movements, progressive frequency increases.Gaining large and small amounts of space (particularly when alternating) and making directional changes and arced runs can be implemented without major organizational effort and easily made a part of training.

The jump rope can also be used as a marker to jump over. When folding the rope and pulling it apart from both ends, it can be used for tuck jumps.

Poles—wooden or plastic—also work well as markers or obstacles at practice. Players can jump over them. For youth players, in particular, the use of ropes as obstacles on the ground is preferable to poles. Landing on a pole often results in sudden sliding. The movement can no longer be controlled, and injury risk increases considerably.

The following are some organizational forms meant to exemplify the use of ropes and poles as obstacles during training. The checks indicate participating players, and the broken lines and black arrows indicate the direction of movement. The triangular markings and black bars indicate ropes or poles are used (see fig. 59).

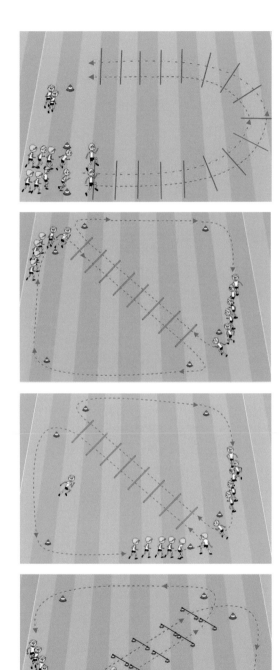

Fig. 59: Six self-explanatory organizational forms for jumping over ropes and poles during team practice

Photos 68 and 69 show two organizational forms in which players are used as important helpers for their teammates. These forms not only serve the practical implementation of motor skill training goals but also the development of joint responsible action, cooperation, and helping and safeguarding each other (team spirit).

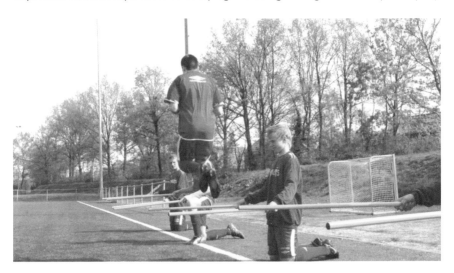

Photo 68: Double-leg jumps over two raised poles

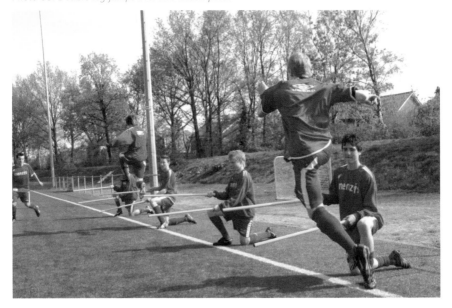

Photo 69: Vertical leaps as in "show jumping" with the help of a partner

14.4   JUMPING EXERCISES WITH MINI HURDLES

The mini hurdle (at different heights) plays an important role in today's jump training because it is a versatile methodological aid that reproduces, in particular, stopping and accelerating distances that constantly occur in modern soccer: single-leg and double-leg jumps during and after duels (on the ground and especially in the air), the foot coming down quickly just below the center of gravity (with little support), and incomplete knee extensions with high stride frequency and long strides during sprints to and away from the ball (Schmidtbleicher, 1984; Mann, 1999). Together with the development of demand-specific overall body tension (see chapter 16), timely initiation, and completion of momentum-generating elements (arms, legs, head, and trunk), training with mini hurdles to achieve a modern sprinting technique in soccer contributes to the ability to successfully execute movements under time pressure.

However, during regular training with players, the authors noticed that multiple jumps over mini hurdles are often just "reeled off." It means that the necessary quality of movement is not always a priority in training when handling time pressure during movements with short action times (development of short time programs) and abrupt strength increase (explosive power). Particularly in youth training, the final push-off, thus the basic finalacceleration program, plays a critical role in speed development with and without the ball, because it only comes into effect at the highest movement speed. Therefore, a high degree of movement quality is crucial to the desired capability of timely and synchronized activation of the fast-twitch muscle fibers, in particular. In modern soccer training, technique and power training are siblings and in terms of speed trainingshould be revamped, as is documented in the following examples for practicaltraining (Voss et al., 2007, p. 32f and 43f). In the "reel-off mode," a high implementation rate of the target movement is always more important than a high loading volume.

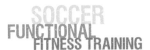
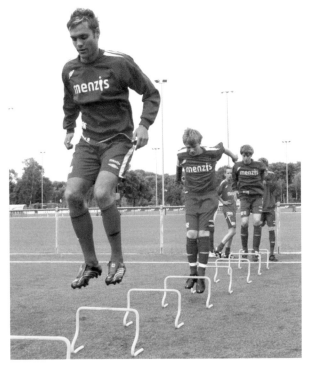

Photo 70: Double-leg jumps over mini hurdles

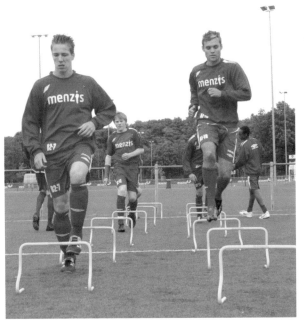

Photo 71: Single-leg jumps in a particular jumping rhythm

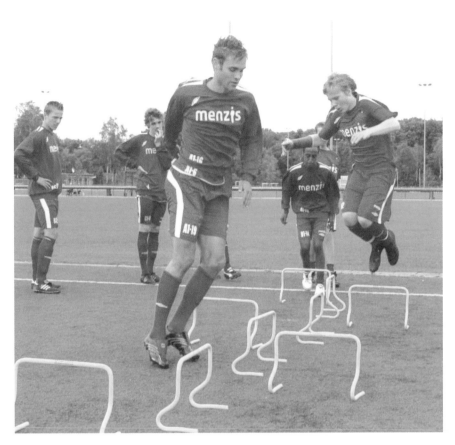

Photo 72: Double-leg jumps with 90-degree turns

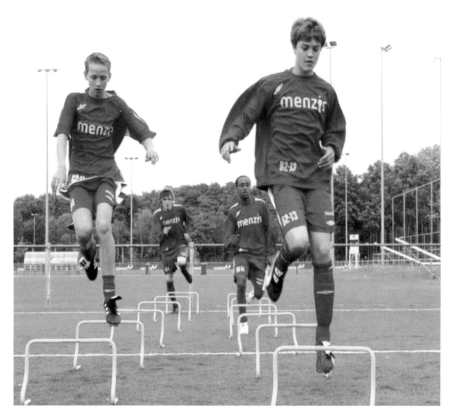

Photo 73: High-knee skips over mini hurdles

High-knee skips constantly alternate the left and right leg over the mini hurdles. For U17/U16 youth players, the distance between hurdles is approximately 10 to 12 feet.

> CHAPTER

15

15 WHY SHOULD SOCCER PLAYERS TURN TO THROWING GAMES?

"The new approach = focus on requirements instead of abilities."

(Roth, Memmert, and Schubert, 2006, p. 37)

In today's modern soccer, continued possession of one's team increasingly depends on the goal player. Using the example of the currently best goal player in the world, Manuel Neuer (FC Bayern Munich), it is evident how critical his throwing technique and function can be for the team and for the implementation of a playing philosophy. When Neuer rapidly transitioned to *offensive action* after intercepting crosses, he was able to greatly accelerate the entire team's game with his precise, long throw-outs of, at times, more than 60 meters, thus putting physical and mental pressure on the opposing team.

A throw from the goal player can, therefore, be considered a type of pass, as these passes (rolling the ball, sidearm throw, overhand throw) send the same message to the teammates as those played by foot. Moreover, a pass by hand can be considerably more accurate than one played by foot, and the ball cannot be stolen as long as the goal player holds it with his hands. Therefore, the execution is not subject to time pressure, which greatly improves the success rate.

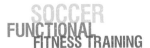

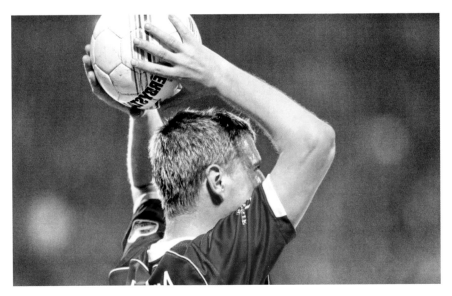

Photo 74: An effective throw-in must be learned!

Furthermore, when taking a look at the number of throw-ins by field players during an average Bundesliga game, it must be noted that there are approximately 50 per game, meaning throw-ins take place on average more often than every two minutes. Throw-ins occur even more frequentlyin competitive youth play since ball control and passing techniques in particular are usually not as precise and reliable, and the ball, therefore, goes into touch more frequently.[22] Since the *throw-in pass* is the only pass in soccer that can be played by hand, it is generally not given much consideration during soccer training: "Anyone can do a throw-in! Both feet on the ground and hands and ball behind the head, that's it."

But here the authors would like to elaborate on some technical and tactical details that coaches and instructors should be aware of and that (next to the goal player's game) argue for more comprehensive and intensive throwing practice as a foundation for a successful *throw-in pass*:

---

22   *With the aid of their mini football academy, Roth, Roth, and Hegar (2014, p. 155-192) effectively demonstrate how to address these important demands on soccer players at an early stage.*

⟡ The thrower is in possession *(passing philosophy)*.

⟡ During the *throw-in pass*, the opponent is in the *majority on the field*, which might seem trivial here, and the team in possession is *outnumbered*. At that moment in the action, many players are not always aware of this fact.

⟡ Is the opposition organized or unorganized in the space? The timing of the *throw-in pass* and whether to throw fast or slow depend on this decision *(passing tactics)*.

⟡ *Throw-in passes* must be precise *(passing technique)*.

⟡ To the teammates, nearly every *throw-in pass* is a waist-high ball that must first be controlled with technical precision (ball control technique).

Moreover, *long throw-in passes*, particularly into the opposing danger zone, can be an effective means for creating a goal-scoring opportunity with a cross using a throw-in near the goal (Hyballa and te Poel, 2015). In addition, a reliable, precise, and dynamic throwing technique depends on good trunk stability. The authors will elaborate on this in subsequent chapters.

Coaches and instructors should, therefore, offer throwing games to all players, particularly in youth soccer (gaining throwing experience) and stress the functional and proper execution[23] of techniques during training (foot placement, body tension, release points, elbow position). Coaches and instructors must exercise preventative measures.

---

23   *Due to the limited scope of this publication, the authors refer to the valid throw-in rules of soccer. These can be viewed at www.fifa.com.*

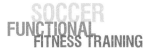
EXERCISE 1: SPEED RACE

Players from two teams (X and O) form a circle together (see fig. 60). Each team has a ball (e.g., soccer ball or medicine ball). At a starting signal from the coach or instructor, both balls are thrown clockwise or counterclockwise from the starting point, using either the left or right hand or with both arms (see photo 75). See which team overtakes the other.

The size of the teams and the circle, the distance between players, the weight of the ball, and the number of rounds and breaks should be chosen so the own team's throwing (and running) can become appropriate for the competition.

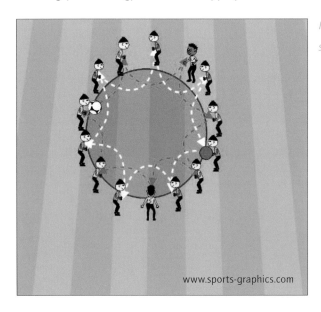

Fig. 60: Speed race with staggered positions

www.sports-graphics.com

VARIATIONS:

- Trailing actions: The player who threw the ball follows his throw and takes the catcher's place. When the last player of each team catches the ball, they run to the places where no players remain, and the competition begins again. See which team overtakes the other.
- The player settles the ball, dribbles, and then plays the ball with a lob pass to the next player for a *throw-in pass*.
- The ball is settled and then played with a chest or volley pass to the next player for a *throw-in pass*.
- A combination of headers and *throw-in passes* must be played.

EXERCISE 2: DODGEBALL

Two teams of equal size face each other on a marked field. Two or three balls are used in this game. Players of both teams must tag each other with the balls. This is done by means of a bounce (using ground contact). If successful, the player who was tagged must quickly sit down at the edge of the field. If a player catches an opposing player's throw, the players sitting at the edge of the field can rejoin the game. See which team has the most field players on the field after a certain amount of playing time.

The field size, number of players and balls, the amount of playing time, break lengths, and repetitions depend on the training goal. The ball material should not be able to cause injury.

VARIATIONS:

- The opposing team's player must now be tagged directly. Players can now try out different behaviors (e.g., standing still for different periods of time or feinting).
- Use "blocking players" that are marked with different colors. Team players can briefly stay in their "cover shadow" to protect themselves from the throws.

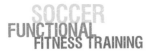
EXERCISE 3: DRIVING BALL

Two teams stand facing each other outside of a marked field. Both teams have several tennis balls and must try to hit a medicine ball placed in the center of the field in order to drive it across a predetermined marker. For every successful team effort (i.e., the medicine ball rolled across the marker), the respective team receives a bonus point. Tennis balls that are left on the field can be retrieved and thrown again. The balls can only be thrown from the own baseline. Rule violations result in penalties (fairness first!). See which team is the first to score three bonus points.

The distance from the medicine ball to the throwers depends on the performance level.

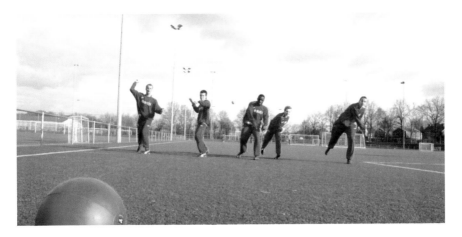

Photo 76: Driving ball: Good aim is key!

VARIATIONS:

- ❯ Do the main exercise but with different support bases (e.g., benches, mini goals). Vary heights.
- ❯ Do the main exercise but with different ball materials.
- ❯ Complete the main exercise but with both arms and *throw-in passes*.
- ❯ Doing the main exercise, use goal player-specific techniques (e.g., rolling, sidearm, overhead).
- ❯ Do the main exercise, but some teammates throw in the balls (e.g., light youth soccer balls) from the sides so the players can play them in the direction of the medicine balls using headers or volley passes.

EXERCISE 4: GAINING SPACE

Two teams stand facing each other on a large field. Players of both teamsare numbered. Number one of the first team throws the medicine ball toward the opposing team (see exercise 3 for team positioning). Number one of that team must throw the ball from where it touched the ground, and so on. Playing time depends on the training goal and performance level. It is important that players get to throw often, take turns quickly, and motivation and effort remain high.

See which team gains the most space within a specified time limit.

VARIATIONS:
- Use different types of balls.
- Use both arms and *throw-in passes*.
- Use goal player-specific techniques (e.g., rolling the ball, sidearm throw, overhead throw).

EXERCISE 5: REBOUND BALL WITH TEAMWORK

Three players are marked with ribbon or bibs of the same color.These playerswork as a team to tag individual players on a marked field with a rebounding ball. They can use only one ball. The three players are not allowed to run with the ball but must try to prepare successful actions using *throw-in passes*. If a player is tagged, he receives a penalty point, but he can continue to play. See how many players the group of three was able to tag during a specified time period.See which player received the fewest penalty points.

The number of evading players and the size of the field depend on the training goal.

VARIATION:
- See exercise 4.

EXERCISE 6: BOUNCE BALL

Form two teams of approximately six players each and issue two balls. The playing area is the size of a volleyball court. It is divided with rows of benches, cones, or mini goals or a tennis net or magic cord into two fields of equal size. By playing (flat) rebounding balls from their field, the two teams try to position the balls so they hit the ground on the opposing field after bouncing on their own field. The opposing team tries to prevent the bouncing balls from hitting the ground on their field by attempting to catch them. See which team scores the most hits.

VARIATION:

❯ See exercise 4.

EXERCISE 7: OVERHEAD BALL

Form two teams (e.g., 3-on-3, as shown in photo 77) and let them compete against each other with two light medicine balls on a marked field (e.g., volleyball court). The two teams are separated by a net (e.g., volleyball net) or a moveable soccer goal. Players from both teams try to throw the medicine ball over the net, using predetermined throwing techniques (e.g., thrust with one or two arms, *throw-in pass*, or throw the medicine ball sideways). If the medicine balls touch the ground, the opposing team receives a bonus point.

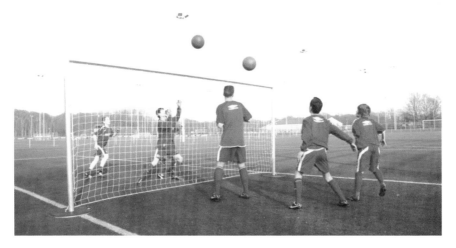

Photo 77: Playing overhead balls as a team

VARIATION:

◉   After a player has thrown the medicine ball over the net, he must leave the field with a quick acceleration to then rejoin play on the field. Coaches or instructors can also set up cones off the fields. Players must then touch or run around these after a throw or thrust. Different color cones can also be used. After a throw or thrust, the coach or instructor calls out the color the player must run to (orientation under time pressure). Teammates should always try to change their positions so they are able to effectively cover the field temporarily while outnumbered (teamwork).

EXERCISE 8: STRESS BALL

Form two teams (see photo 78 with two teams of 10 players each). One team, numbered 1 through 10, sits in a line on a bench or on the ground. The second team is spread out on a marked field. Number one of the seated team throws a medicine ball onto the field and then continuously runs around his own team, clockwise or counterclockwise. For each round, the player scores a point. In the meantime, the team on the field tries to catch the medicine ball and then quickly lines up behind the catcher in a straddle position. The medicine ball is then passed to the next player through the legs. This player accepts the medicine ball and then hands it forward overhead to the next player. The medicine ball is, thus, transferred in a wave. Once the medicine ball reaches the last player, he shouts "Stop!" The coach or instructor asks for the number of rounds that have been run and continues the game with the number two player, and so on. Once all players have a turn, the points are added up and recorded. Then tasks change. See which team is best able to get organized or run the fastest. Here we recommend using a reward system: The team workers of the day are exempt from clean-up, for example.

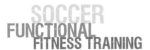

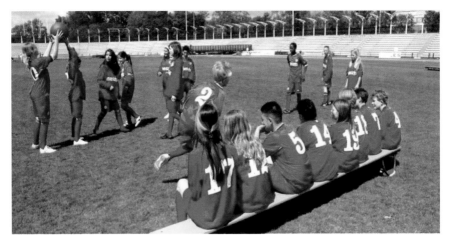

Photo 78: Teamwork against speed

VARIATIONS:

- Form smaller teams—for example, backfour against the forward line or midfielders against wing players.
- Each sprinter sits down after running one round and another teammate takes over.

EXERCISE 9: PRECISION RULES!

Players stand approximately 20 meters apart with cone markers set up between them (see photo 79). Players try to hit the cones with handballs, tennis balls, softballs, or soccer balls. See which player is the first to score three hits.

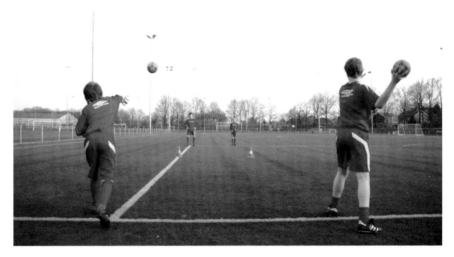

Photo 79: Precise throwing can't be taken for granted. Practice makes perfect!

VARIATIONS:

- Set up several cones on a bench. See which player clears the cones off the bench fastest with overhead throws. Precision and speed are a must here!
- Use both arms and *throw-in passes*.
- Add a third player who flicks a volley, header, or chest pass on the second player.
- Use goal player-specific techniques (rolling the ball, sidearm throw, overhead throw).
- Perform exercise in a gym with swinging ropes.
- Use a different formation, such as triangle, diamond, five- or six-row grids (Hyballa and te Poel, 2015).

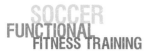
EXERCISE 10: ACROBATS

Players place a ball in the large opening of a cone and then use the cone to toss the ball high into the air. After a dynamic whole-body extension, try to catch the ball softly with the cone (see photo 80). See which player catches the most balls within a specified time period. Specify a minimum height for throws.

It can be marked on a fence or soccer pendulum unit, visible to all.

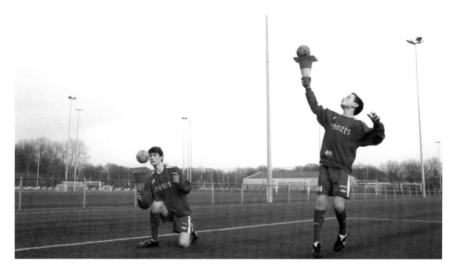

Photo 80: The soccer player as acrobat

VARIATIONS:

- Use different types of balls and different size cones.
- Use two cones per player.
- Use multiple balls per player.
- Use both arms.
- Incorporate different rolling exercises (e.g., forward or backward roll or to the side) after whole-body extension.
- Do the main exercise as a partner exercise (trade balls).
- Incorporate solving math problems.

EXERCISE 11: CATCHER

Form groups of five: three throwers and two catchers (see photo 81). The two catchers use a net they make themselves (in photo 81, a gymnastics hoop with a net) and stand side by side at a specified distance. The throwers take turns trying to throw the ball overhead into the net from a marked spot. See which team scores the most points within a certain amount of time. Cooperation and communication are very important here. There should be a sufficient number of balls.

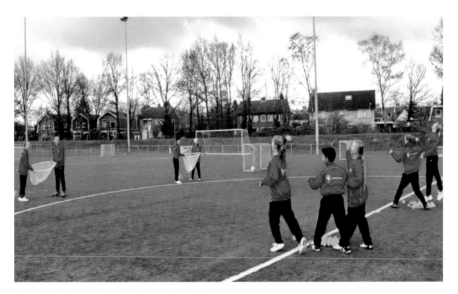

Photo 81: Communal throwing and catching

VARIATIONS:

- See exercise 10.
- The group stands at the starting point, and the throwers throw the balls into the path of the catchers. See which team can throw farthest without the ball touching the ground.

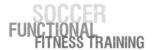
EXERCISE 12: SKEWERING RINGS

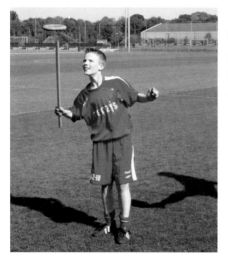

Pairs of players stand facing each other approximately 10 meters apart. They attempt to toss and catch a rubber ring back and forth with a stick or baton. See which pair scores the most points.

Photo 82: Find the ring's center.

VARIATIONS:

- ❯ Use both arms.
- ❯ Use different size rings, sticks, and batons.
- ❯ Moving target: The partner is in motion.
- ❯ Permanently increase or decrease distances.
- ❯ Increase the height of the throw and, thus, the amount of effort (e.g., throw over soccer goals or magic cords).
- ❯ Add a third player. He tries to interfere with the throw (actively or somewhat actively).

CHAPTER

16

16 STRENGTH AND ATHLETIC TRAINING IN YOUTH SOCCER

"The difference between youth players and senior players is obvious in nearly every aspect. However, (takeoff) power performancesthat have been measured show no evidence of pro players being dominant over youth players who do strength training. This makes clear that strength training can apparently neutralize age-specific performance differences in the stretch-shortening cycle (SSC). According to this long-term, periodized strength training is recommended in youth soccer in order to ease the entry into senior soccer."

(Sander et al., 2013, p. 24)

Since movements in soccer are mostly dynamic and highly explosive and can be characterized by accelerating or decelerating manifestations of strength, trained coaches and instructors are urged to pay attention to the development of musculature during training that is both powerful and has endurance and to not neglect static work.

In chapters 7, 8, and 9, the authors point out that in the future an increased integration of strength and athletic training into a performance-enhancing and preventative overall training concept in elite sports-oriented youth soccer as well as in high-level amateur soccer is recommended (Lopez-Segova et al., 2010; Silvestre et al., 2006; Javanovic et al., 2011). In confirmation of this assertion, the authors briefly reference, in no particular order, the following study results:

- In their studies,Hoff (2005), Masuda et al. (2005), Weineck (2004), and Wisloff et al. (2004) show that the importance of *maximum strength in thelower extremities* in particular is critical to powerful movements such as sprints, jumps, or shots on goal in soccer.

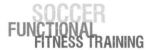

❯ In the course of researching quantitative methods for performance diagnostics in competitive soccer, Broich (2009) was able to focus particularly on the isometric and dynamic strength of performance-determining muscles and muscle groups and was, thus, able to focus on how to outline the optimal agonist to antagonist ratio (balance). Broich emphasized that "there is a significant link between maximum isometric and dynamic strength of knee flexors and knee extensors and the power and maximum performance capacity in pro soccer players. The level of dynamic strength of knee flexors and extensors influences the quality of relative strength and power-based movements" (p. 41). Furthermore, while conducting measurements in the knee extensor area, Broich found that there are significant differences in the level of dynamic strength between pro and youth players (p. 47). From this, Broich deduced that the *knee extensor's level of dynamic strength* is increasingly important during competition as a critical factor in maximally accelerated movements. Moreover, it can be assumed that there is a correlation between maximum dynamic strength in isokinetic measurements of the knee extensors and ball velocity during shots (Newman et al., 2004, p. 867-872; Masuda et al., 2005, p. 44-52).

❯ Next to maximum strength, developing reactive strength for jumping and speed-related performance is extremely important in soccer (Güllich, 1996; Cometti et al., 2001; Schlumberger, 2006; Kollath et al., 2006; Kotzamanidis et al., 2005). Power-oriented maximum strength weight training should be a standard concomitant activity to *reinforce reactive strength* in soccer players (Broich, 2009, p. 49).

❯ "*The maximum isometric strength* of knee extensors and flexors is of fundamental importance to explosive strength as well as maximum dynamic strength. The main goal is to facilitate an optimized training-induced improvement of performance-limiting factors in soccer by identifying individual strengths and weaknesses" (Broich, 2009, p. 51).

❯ "The game of soccer is largely comprised of very one-sided muscle loading. This results in one-sided muscular strength development in the working muscles, and the neglect of the antagonist muscles as well as the stabilizing (red) muscles" (Broich, 2009, p. 52).

- Studies by Caldwell et al. (2009) and La Torre et al. (2007) document that soccer trainingexclusively during the season does not result in improved sprinting and jumping performance (also see Ronnestad et al., 2008, and Ronnestad et al., 2011).

- Lockie et al. obtained empirical evidence that strength training can result in a higher sprint performance increaseover 5 to 10 meters than sprint training.

- Sander et al. (2012) found that it is possible to integrate strength training twice a week as part of a comprehensive training concept in youth soccer, and that it can lead to performance increases in, for instance, U15/U14 players over 30-meter sprint distances (p. 42).

- Rowland (2004) points out that it can be assumed that *10-year long-term and versatile (and periodized)* strength training will contribute to developing a good sprint performance.

- In a study with elite youth athletes, Ullrich et al. (2014) were able to show that even just 10-week concomitant strength-endurance training resulted in systematic adaptations of the neuromuscular fatigue resistance of trunk extensor and flexor muscles and moderate increases of MVC[24] in the major muscle groups. In this context, Myer et al. (2008) already linked limited neuromuscular capacities of large trunk muscle groups to injuries to the ACL in female athletes, and Weineck (2004, p. 203) attributes typical "back pain" in soccer to weak stomach and back muscles.

- The Dutch professional goalie trainer Eddie Pasveer (formerly with FC Twente Enschede and De Graafschap) developed an innovative functional approach using the well-known Varioelastic band for the athletic training of goal players and is very successful with this method. Due to publication limits, we will at this time only reference the DVD (epasveer@home.nl).

---

24 *MVC stands for maximum voluntary contraction. In a muscle, this is usually calculated through median amplitude of the highest signal portion.*

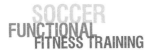

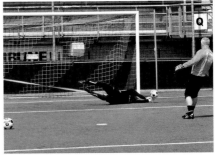

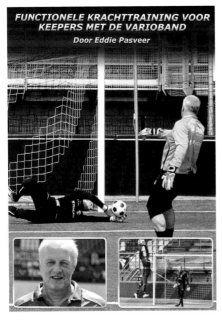

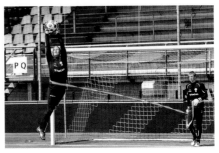

Photo 83: Eddie Pasveer during professional goal player training with the Varioband (epasveer@ home.nl)

"Five units per week. In addition we visit the weight room three times a week. Youth soccer games are already very physical. The tackles are really different than in Germany."

(Yusuf Coban, age 18, born in Aalen, Germany, and U18/U19 player for the Premier League clubs Stoke City, in a kicker 24 interview from March 16, 2015, 24, p. 22)

In summary, the use of different training means for the purpose of, for instance, developing power results in a performance increase and can be simplified and outlined as follows:

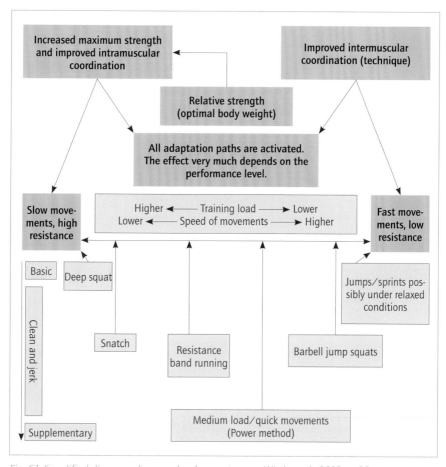

Fig. 61: Simplified diagram of power development as per Wirth et al., 2012, p. 38

As discussed in chapter 1, in modern soccer training, a lot of attention should be focused on athletic training as a form of soccer fitness within the long-term training process. Depending on age and stage of development, this is supplemented with classic strength training using free weights and modern fitness studio and special developmental equipment and is geared primarily toward the optimization of a pro soccer player's most important abilities of maximum and explosive strength.[25] Training with high intensity loads and the goal of optimal power displacement (Wirth et al., 2012, p. 36-42) presupposes extensive and detailed knowledge, particularly about training with free weights, and licensed soccer coaches and

---

25   *Strength training that is characterized by major muscle contractions is the crucial trigger for the release of titin kinase from the contractile protein titin, which ultimately triggers muscle hypertrophy (Hottenrott and Neumann, 2010, p. 13).*

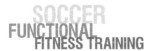

instructors should combine this with an additional sports science degree, as well as coaching courses through the U.S. Soccer Federation's national coaching schools.[26] The topic of classic strength training will, therefore, not be discussed hereafter.[27] This also applies to stretching, warm-ups, cool-downs, and the periods of time for adaptation processes, periodization, and regeneration before[28] and after a game and practice for soccer players.

The following points shall be summed up for (1) the method of stretching and (2) training planning in soccer training (cp. Freiwald, 2009, p. 288-297):

1. All stretching methods lead to a better joint mobility. The most effective ones are CR-AC, AC, DS, CR and SS.
2. The individual goal of stretching has to be determined before. A sustainable development of flexibility involves independent training sessions. Determining standard load norms as well as writing training protocols are absolutely necessary.

Here the authors refer the readers to existing relevant sources that address this important topic for training and competition in detail and in a practice-oriented manner: Wegmann (2012), Timmermanns (2010), Freiwald (2009), and Oltmanns (2009).

The former select coach for the Hessian soccer association, Günter Wegmann, was able to combine both subject areas in a DVD on stretching and strengthening for soccer players from the angle of a long-term performance buildup and preventative action by the coach or instructor using targeted and systematic soccer training. We will, therefore, purposely relinquish this interface at this point.

---

26 *Current barbell training at the Training Academies in Cologne, Germany, includes 96 learning units over four months/blocks (plus in-depth work of approximately 20 learning units with the own players). Furthermore, a training term paper that provides the basis for a theoretical exam is required. Training concludes with a certification.*

27 *At this point, we refer the interested reader to the current debate about the value of barbell training in game sports at different performance levels (Steinhöfer, 2014). It goes into the currently unresolved question of how the bilateral transfer mechanisms of motor abilities actually function (Issurin, 2013).*

28 *At this point, we will reference current published works on the subjects of fatigue and regeneration in the magazine* **Leistungssport** *(2014, 44(5)). In this respect the enzyme mTORC1 (protein complex component) during the formation of proteins after strength training (up to six hours) appears to be particularly important to the anticipated adaptation processes (training design: see Schnur, 2014, p. 97).*

When planning, implementing, and evaluating a strength and athletic training program, it is still extremely important for the coach or instructor to be able to assess the training group and each individual player with respect to strength, overall teamwork within the group, and knowledge about safeguarding and assisting. To highlight some general strategies within the scope of a multi-year performance buildup, particularly with respect to strength, we will hereafter present a chart of exemplary and not sport-oriented key parameters of process-oriented training.

*Table 12: Multi-year buildup of maximum strength and power (*subject to the sport's demand profile and the training period) as per Wirth et al., 2012, p. 45*

Multi-year buildup of maximum strength and power				
Stage of development	Volume	Intensity	Duration	Goal
Start of strength training	Low	Low	One year	Technical skills
General strength training	Moderate	Moderately low	Two years	Developing physiological foundations/technical skills
Start of targeted strength development	Moderately high*	Moderately high*	Three years	Developing high quality of movements during training exercises Beginning of sport-specific development of physiological characteristics
Development of maximum strength*	High*	Maximally high*		Developing highest quality of movement during training exercises Maximum development of physiological characteristics*

In strength and athletic training, the prevention of accidents must be a top priority. When starting long-term strength and athletic training (see chapter 8), the authors recommend testing procedures (including measuring instruments) that are now available for ambitious soccer training.Because extensive detail exceeds the scope of this book, the authors reference the following sources consisting of copious reports from internal medicine studies, immune status analyses, orthopedic trauma studies, diagnostics of biomechanical functions, differential diagnostics of

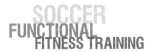

endurance and strength, and soccer-specific technical-coordinated study designs: Beck &Bös (1995, p. 209-251); McGill et al., (1999 and 2002); Beck et al. (2006, p. 151-158); Durastani and Durastani (2008); Kleinöder (2004, p. 58-65); Lottermann, Laudenklos, and Friedrich (2003, p. 6-15); Mester and Kleinöder (2008, p. 27-48); Weineck (2004, p. 329-346); and Swiss Olympic (2003).

In the subsequent chapters, we will, therefore, proceed according to the variational principle when choosing training content and execution modalities (with stable or unstable support surfaces) and link this content with elements of team building and group and team leadership. Here the authors make sure that the reader is able to draw on movement patterns and devices during practice that make the use of machines (including cable machines) unnecessary at this point (resource-based economy).[29]

For pre-puberty strength and athletic training, the following recommendations should be taken into account:

Table 13: Recommendations on pre-puberty strength and athletic training borrowing from Wirth et al., 2012, p. 45

Training stage	Sets	Repetitions	Adaptation
Base	3	10-15	Neuronal/morphological
Strength	3	6-10	Neuronal/morphological
Power	2-3	6-8	Neuronal
Peaking	1-2	6-8	Neuronal
Aktive Pause	−	−	−

---

29 At this time, we simply reference current fitness trends in athletic training for soccer, such as Cross Fit (Beilenhoff, 2015, p. 18-27).

16.1 ATHLETIC TRAINING IN GAME FORM

EXERCISE 1: HANDS UP AND SPEED!

Several groups of approximately five players play against each other. Five youth players sit one behind the other, and at a signal from the coach or instructor, the front player (number one) passes the medicine ball overhead to the player behind him. Then he quickly stands up and runs to the rear of his group and sits down. Player two repeats this process, and so on. In doing so, the group shifts backwards.

The weight of the medicine ball should be chosen based on training level and training emphasis.

COMPETITION RULES:

- ❯ See which group is fastest to move a specified distance.

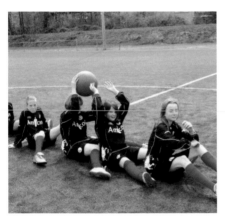 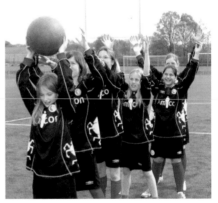

Photo 84: Passing a medicine ball down the line   *Photo 85: Passing the medicine ball overhead down the line and then rolling it back to the front through thelegs*

VARIATION:

- ❯ Complete the main exercise standing (photo 85).

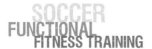
EXERCISE 2: THROW-IN RELAY

Form two groups of five youth players each and ask them to position themselves in the order shown in photo 86. The goal is to throw the medicine ball to the teammate with a proper throw. Sequence: Player 1 (on right) throws the medicine ball to player 2 (on left), who throws it back to player 1 and then crouches back down. Player 1 then throws to player 3, and so on. After player 5 throws the medicine ball to player 1, he takes over his position. Now player 1 stands in front of player 2. The weight of the medicine ball should be chosen based on training level and training emphasis.

COMPETITION RULE:

◎ See which group is the first to completely trade places.

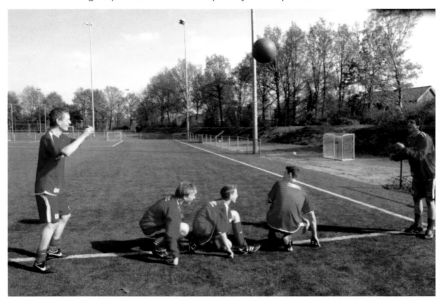

Photo 86: Team spirit and timing during the throw-in relay

EXERCISE 3: WILL THE BRIDGE HOLD?

Groups of five players each form a bridge (see photo 87) and must roll a medicine ball back and forth below the bridge.

COMPETITION RULE:

❂ See which group is the quickest to roll the medicine back and forth eight times.

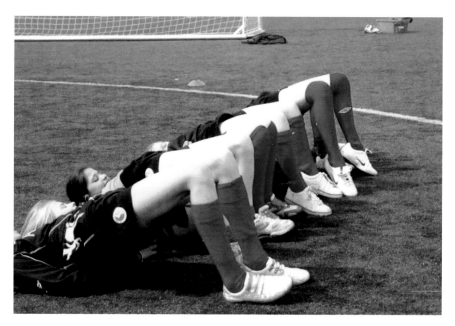

Photo 87: The bridge must maintain tension!

VARIATION:

❂ Three players get into push-up position, lifting their trunks so the ball can roll through underneath. Two players roll the ball back and forth eight times from the head end. Competition rule: Same as main exercise but change tasks.

The number of repetitions and series and the weight of the medicine ball should be chosen based on the group's training level and the training goal.

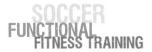
EXERCISE 4: PASS THE PACKAGE!

Form groups of equal size and pass the medicine ball forward and back as shown in photo 88. Legs must be in straddle position. The back player (and subsequently all players) must make a half turn after receiving the medicine ball and then pass the medicine ball, which cannot touch the ground, back from the opposite side.

COMPETITION RULE:

◈   See which group is the fastest after, for instance, eight rounds. If the ball falls to the ground, it must be returned to the start.

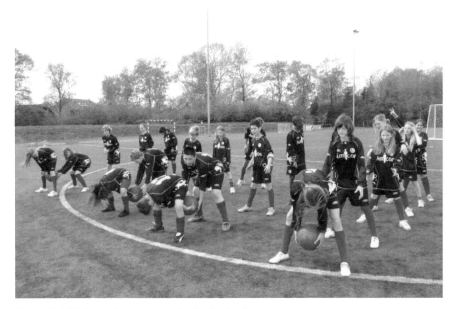

Photo 88: Will the package arrive at its destination?

EXERCISE 5: BENCH LIFTING

Determine group sizes based on the size and weight of available benches and the performance level and training goal.Have the players first practice the coordinated technical process of lifting the bench several times (see photo 89, a-b). One player in the group, and if possible every player in the group, should have this responsibility during the course of the exercise: The player announces the start of the joint lifting process, and the coach or instructor ensures the safe execution (safeguarding and assisting). Once the process is completed safely and cooperatively, the following competition rule can be implemented: See which group is quickest to transport the bench back and forth six times. The number of series depends on the performance level and training goal.

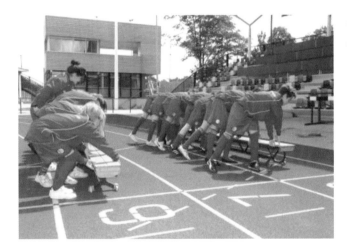

Photo 89a: Teamwork is key!

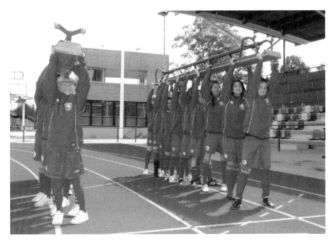

Photo 89b: Lifting overhead and safely setting down on the other side

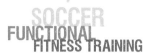
EXERCISE 6: REVERSE GEAR

See exercise 5in which the groups must jointly pass the bench backwards through their legs so, as per the competition rules, (1) it does not touch the ground, (2) the front player always runs to the rear of the group after he finishes lifting (and holds on to the bench again there), and (3) the entire bench must be transported across a line (marker).

The distance to the line depends on performance level and training goal.

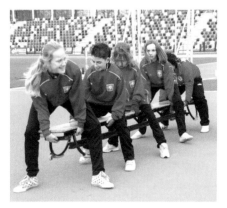

Photo 90a: Static effort, teamwork, and dexterity are key!

Photo 90b: Thrust and dexterity, a demanding team effort!

VARIATIONS:

- Pass the bench forward.
- Pass the bench forward overhead (see photo 90b). Caution: The bench cannot touch the head or the sequence has to start over. Use the arms as buffers.

EXERCISE 7: WE WILL SUPPORT AND HOLD YOU!

See exercise 6 in which players must hold the bottom of the bench with their arms at head level so the player is able to closely watch the process. One teammate balances from one end to the other. A "mount" (vaulting boxes) with spotters on either side (teammate on the left and right) is recommended to initially make balancing safer. At the end of the balancing act, the player should jump off the bench and land safely and softly. A soft, dry, and even surface is recommended. The dismount can also be assisted by the two safeguarding teammates. Safeguarding elements from gymnastics or acrobatics should first be practiced thoroughly. (Key words: pinch grip, support grip, and pinch grip in form of a twist grip). Here, too, the principles of cooperation and communication play an important role.

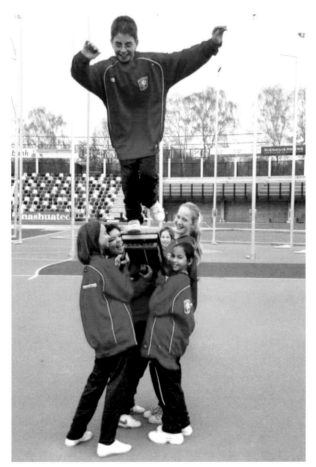

Photo 91a: Strength, courage, and shared responsibility go hand in hand.

VARIATIONS:

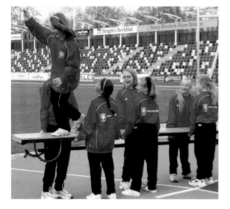

Photo 91b: Holding and balancing as a team.
Mutual trust is everything!

- Have the players jointly lift the bench to hip level using an open grip with palm up (see photo 91b).

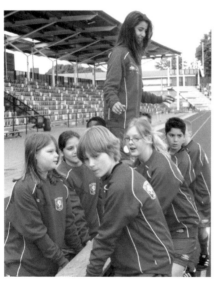

Photo 91c: Holding on tight and finishing together.

- The group must safely and quickly transport a player across a designated marker using a long bench. Compete against other groups for time or on a course (see photo 91c).

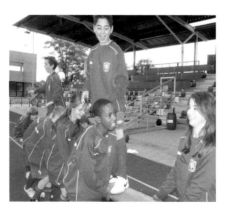

Photo 91d: Responsibility and effort increase.

- Two players are on the bench and are transported. Support points should be designated so weight will be evenly distributed (see photo 91d).

EXERCISE 8: CRAWLER

Form groups of three and let the players crawl backwards while hanging, as shown in photo 92, whereby the pole must be held with a reverse grip. If possible, carriers should hold and carry the poles with a mixed grip (pronated and supinated). Carriers must be instructed not to let go of the poles during transport. Communication among the group of three is absolutely required.

COMPETITION FORMATS:

◉ Depending on performance level and training goal, player groups of three must run around a distant marker (e.g., cone) and return to the starting point. There they switch partners. See which group switches fastest.

◉ Complete main exercise on a course that must be set up.

◉ Complete main exercise as a relay race.

◉ Complete main exercise using a guiding a ball.

◉ Complete main exercise, but in cases of highly developed technical skills, juggle the ball on a course with and without ground contact.

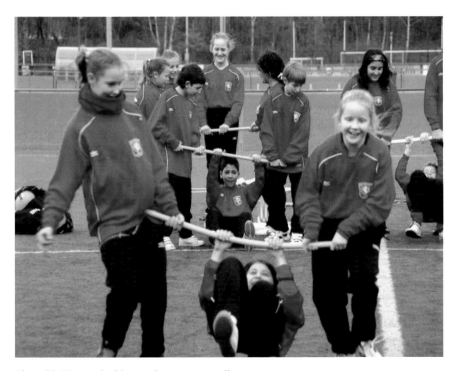

Photo 92: We can do this together at top speed!

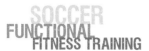

EXERCISE 9: TRANSPORTER

Players execute the formatshown in photo 93 in groups of four, whereby one player must remain in a push-up position. Grips are the same as in exercise 8. The rear carrier safeguards with an adjusted half pinch grip above the ankles.

COMPETITION FORMATS:

❯ See exercise 8.

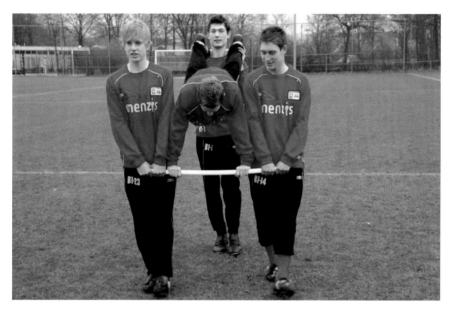

Photo 93: Getting to the finish quickly and safely with lots of body tension and teamwork

EXERCISE 10: BACKWARDS AIRPLANE

Depending on performance level, training emphasis, and bodyweight of the players, form groups that are capable of supporting one player and passing him to the rear as shown in photo 94. The back player then holds the player under both arms with a half pinch grip and,coordinating with his teammates, safely lowers him to the ground.

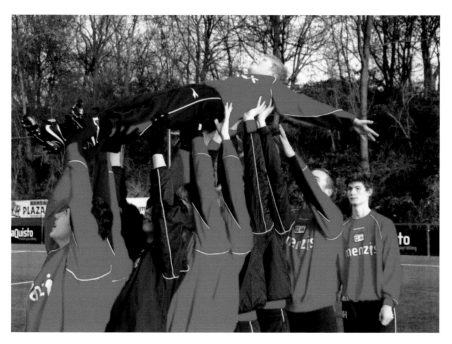

Photo 94: "You can trust us!"

To start this powerful exercise in trust, the player is lifted from a crouch position and then tightens up his entire body with his arms extended to the side. This format can only be executed with players who are able to accurately safeguard and assist and are aware of their great responsibility for the safety of the player they are passing backwards. The coach should double up on spotters, only choose level and dry surfaces, and if possible, lay out soft floor mats on both sidesfor safety. The number of repetitions depends on the training goal.

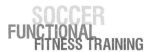

16.2 TRAINING STRENGTH AND BALANCE

In today's soccer, increased strength potential and improved joint stability are basic elements of athletic training (Kollath and Buschmann, 2010, p. 18-19; Ülsmann, 2012). When adapting to different surfaces—old and new artificial turf, grass, cinders, gym floor (Futsal), sand (beach soccer), and different types of plastic coating (outdoor multipurpose facilities)—weather, and intensified dueling action (on the ground, while jumping, and in the air), a lack of balance and stability results especially in increased injury risk and limited complex performance capacity.

The following exercises focus primarily on *proprioceptive*[30] and *sensorimotor*[31] training, whereby the latter can be considered synonymous with today's common term *stabilization training*. From a sport-specific point of view, the goal of static and *dynamic stabilization* is to facilitate the steady and precise execution of movements, injury prevention due to overloading, and post-injury rehabilitation (see p. 15).

---

30 *The four receptors (muscle spindle, joint receptors, tendon spindles, and skin receptors) allow the players to orient themselves in space through the position and movement of their joints.*

31 *Is based on the perception and processing of sensory information (vestibular, acoustic, visual, tactile, and kinesthetic). Proprioception provides the foundation. It takes effect through training during optimization of information reception and processing and the conversion of sensory information to a corresponding movement (**Kollath** and **Buschmann**, 2010, p. 11-14).*

16.2.1 INDIVIDUAL STRENGTH AND BALANCE TRAINING

The following exercises depend on the players' performance level and stage of development as well as the coach's training goals and training emphasis. The authors will, therefore, not offer any specific details or benchmarksregarding the structure of exercise loads. However, the yellow dots in many of the photos are intended to provide the coach with important visual directions for functional and effective training.

The following exercises can be used as part of a warm-up routine in soccer training, basic training between warm-up and the first main component, the main focus within the main component, or as a separate training unit. In addition to the aspects listed in chapter 16.1, it should be modified as follows for the training process: bilateral exercises, with external interference factors, at varying speeds, time pressure, orientation, precision, and complexity (Kröger and Roth, 2014).

EXERCISE 1

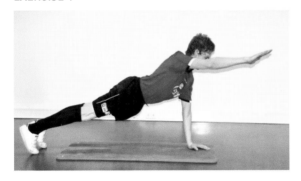

Photo 95: Get into push-up position and alternate arm extension to lengthen the body axis. The hips do not rotate.

EXERCISE 2

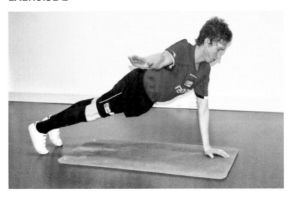

Photo 96: Perform the same as exercise 1, but with alternate arm extension to the side.

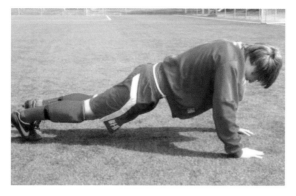

EXERCISE 3

Photo 97: From a push-up position, by quickly pushing off the ground with the hands and landing softly, the player performs a succession of body and arm extensions. It is similar to "hooping" with the arms.

EXERCISE 4

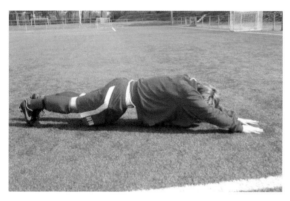

Photo 98: Hold the final position!

EXERCISE 5

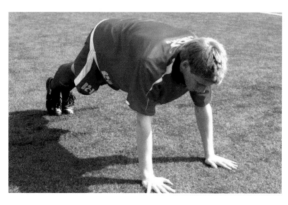

Photo 99: Starting position for the spider (see photo 100).

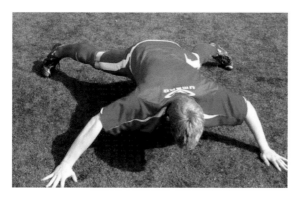

EXERCISE 6

Photo 100: How big can you make the spider? Hold the final position!

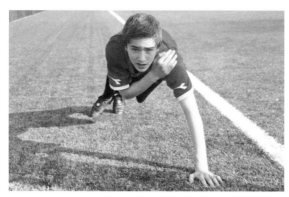

EXERCISE 7

Photo 101: Get into push-up position and alternate bringing each hand to the opposite shoulder.

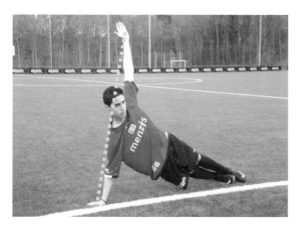

EXERCISE 8

Photo 102: From a push-up position, move into a side plank, alternating sides. The trunk and legs should form a straight line. This also applies to the arm and shoulder alignment.

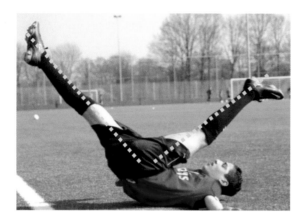

EXERCISE 9

Photo 103: Perform a scissor motion, alternating legs. The angle should not exceed 90 degrees.

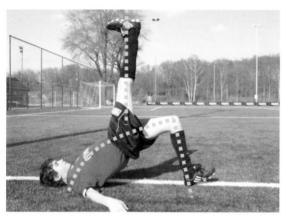

EXERCISE 10

Photo 104: Alternate leg extension from a bridge position. Hips are high!

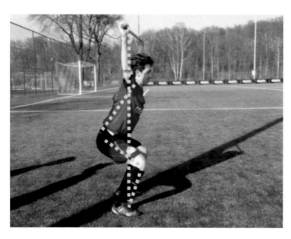

EXERCISE 11

Photo 105: Perform smooth squats with a bar.

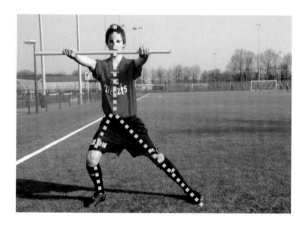

EXERCISE 12

Photo 106: Perform front arm extension with simultaneous alternating side lunge, left and right, with upright trunk position.

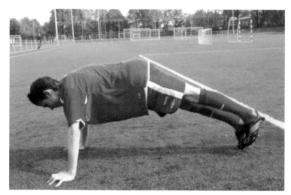

EXERCISE 13

Photo 107: From a push-up position, start to "sag" while extending one leg as high as possible. Alternate legs. (See photo 108.)

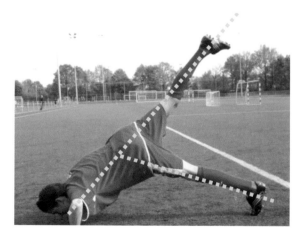

EXERCISE 14

Photo 108: From a low push-up position, extend one leg up high as an extension of the trunk.

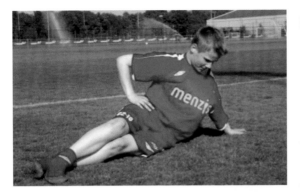

EXERCISE 15

Photo 109: Lying on the side with legs stacked and extended, lift the hip off the ground.

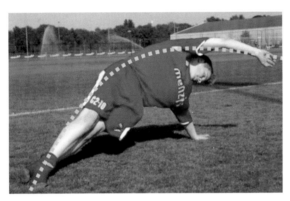

EXERCISE 16

Photo 110: Push off the ground and into an arc with the free arm extended overhead.

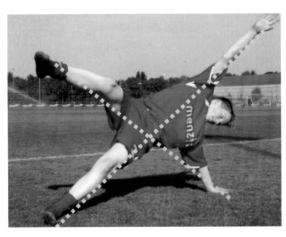

EXERCISE 17

Photo 111: Perform a jumping jack from a full side plank and hold the final position.

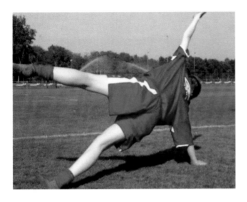

EXERCISE 18

Photo 112: Switch sides and balance (see photo 111).

EXERCISE 19

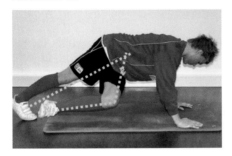
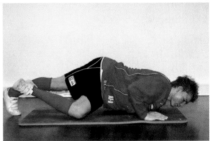

Photo 113, a-b: In a single-leg push-up position, movethe free leg to the inside without touching the floor; the arms are bent and then straightened again.

EXERCISE 20

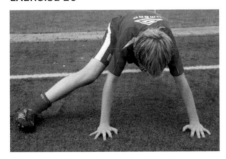
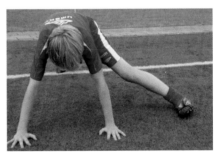

Photo 114, a-b: From a push-up position, jump, alternating sides (left and right).

EXERCISE 21

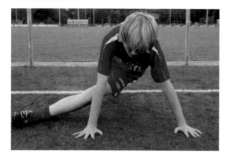 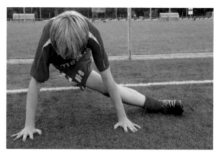

Photo 115, a-b: See photo 114, a-b, in which (rhythmic) jumps are now diagonal followed by a stop, or for advanced athletes, a continual side-to-side scissor motion.

EXERCISE 22

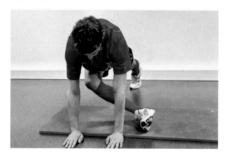 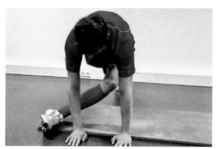

Photo 116, a-b: From a push-up position, perform diagonal alternating jumps. Here the front foot moves to the inside and as close as possible past hands and arms.

EXERCISE 23

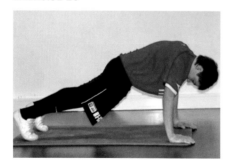 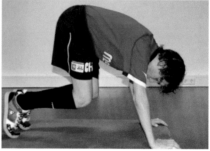

Photo 117, a-b: Perform a squat jump from a push-up position to a 90-degree angle of the knee joint.

EXERCISE 24

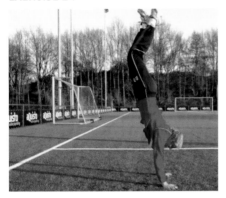 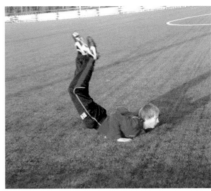

Photo 118, a-b: From a handstand, gradually bend the elbows to roll onto the stomach and then move back into the handstand by dissolving the arching movement of the trunk (ventral). Do this with spotters and instruct them in handholds.

EXERCISE 25

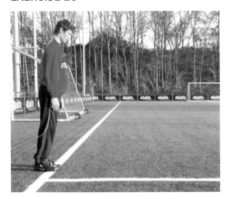 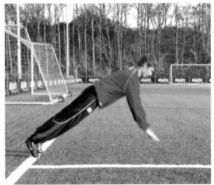

Photo 119, a-b: From a vertical standing position, fall forward like a board, and then softly catch yourself with your arms. Beginners practice from a kneeling position.

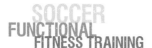
EXERCISE 26

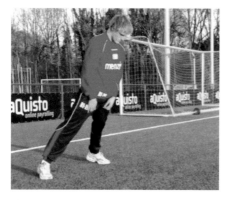
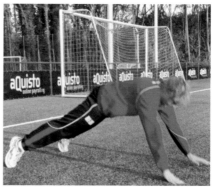

Photo 120, a-b: See photo 119, a-b.This timethe player is in a straddle position.

EXERCISE 27

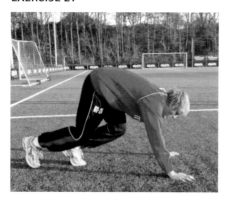
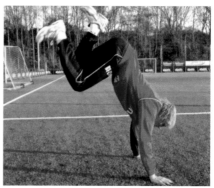

Photo 121, a-b: From the starting position, the player jumps into a near vertical position while maintaining his starting posture, and then lands softly.

EXERCISE 28

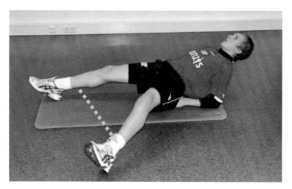

Photo 122: Perform scissor movements of the legs from a reverse elbow plank position.

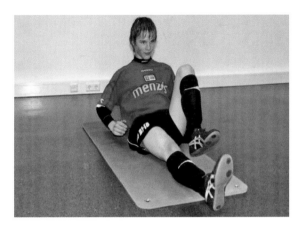

EXERCISE 29

Photo 123: Perform bicycles from a seated position with extended legs.

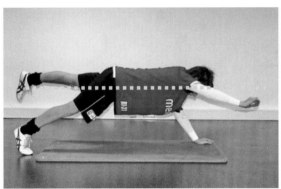

EXERCISE 30

Photo 124: Reciprocal total-body extension in push-up position with time limit.

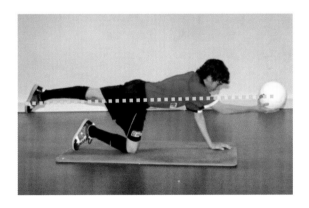

EXERCISE 31

Photo 125: Reciprocal hand and knee balance with ball transfer from one hand to the other.

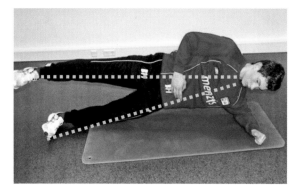

EXERCISE 32

Photo 126: Perform an elbow side plank with raised free leg. Alternate sides.

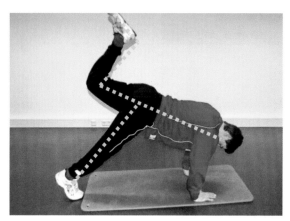

EXERCISE 33

Photo 127: From a pushup position, move one leg into a vertical position with the knee bent to a 90° angle. Alternate legs.

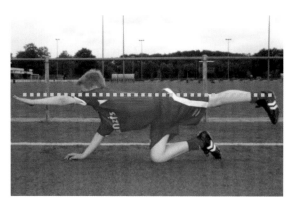

EXERCISE 34

Photo 128: Balance on one hand and one knee on the same side of the body, and alternate sides.

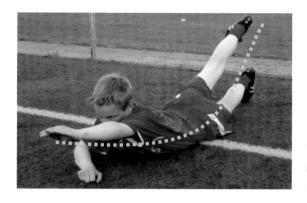

EXERCISE 35

Photo 129: From a prone position, lift opposite arm and leg and hold.

EXERCISE 36

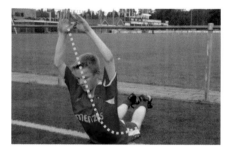

Photo 130a: Bend your trunk into a half-circle.

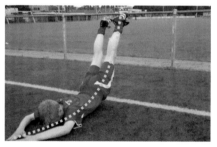

Photo 130b: Extend your trunk in prone position and create a rocking motion.

EXERCISE 37

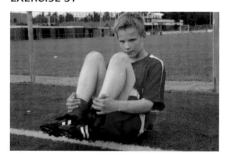

Photo 131a: In a seated position, bend your knees and hold on to your lower legs.

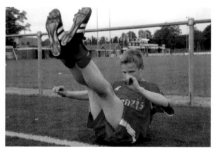

Photo 131b: Extend both legs without falling backwards.

EXERCISE 38

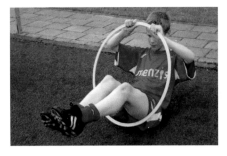 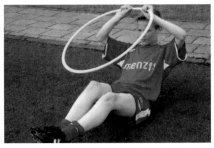

Photo 132a: Extend and bend your legs through the hoop.

Photo 132b: Play with your trunk and balance.

EXERCISE 39

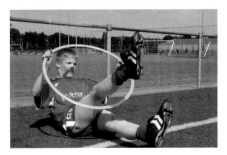 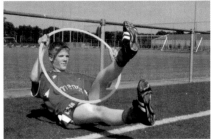

Photo 133a: See exercise 38, but this time the legs alternately move through the hoop.

Photo 133b: Sit up straight and extend your legs.

EXERCISE 40

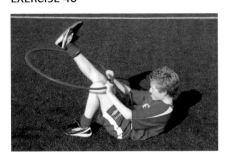 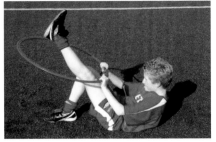

Photo 134a: Alternately extend the left and the right leg through the hoop. One leg always stays on the ground.

Photo 134b: The trunk can touch the ground between leg extensions.

EXERCISE 41

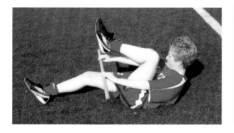 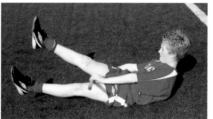

Photo 135a: Alternately extend thelegs over the bar.

Photo 135b: Always extend thelegs all the way and keep thetrunk, creating a belly swing.

EXERCISE 42

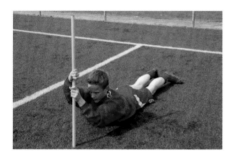 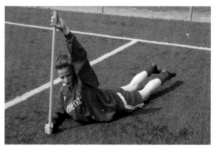

Photo 136a: Hold on to the middle of the bar. Turn it 180 degrees and at the same time lift thetrunk, creating a belly swing.

Photo 136b: Hold on to the ends of the bar. Turn it 180 degrees, righting the body so the trunk is lifted.

EXERCISE 43

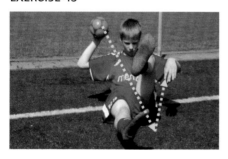 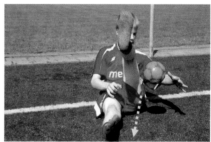

Photo 137a: Balancing on thesit-bones, alternately lift theextended legs and bounce a handball from the inside to the outside.

Photo 137b: Keep thelegs as straight as possible.

EXERCISE 44

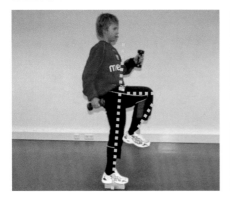

Photo 138a: Stand with one leg on a block and perform a countermovement with knees and arms (with weights at a 90-degree angle).

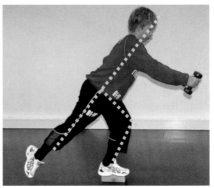

Photo 138b: Now extend one leg back.

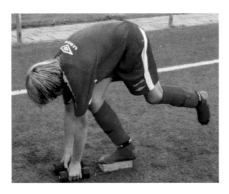

Photo 138c: Touch the weights to the ground.

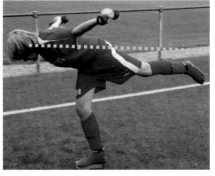

Photo 138d: Move into a standing single-leg balance pose. Trunk and extended leg form a nearly straight line.

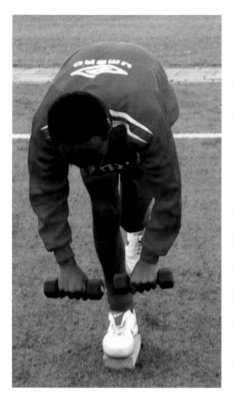 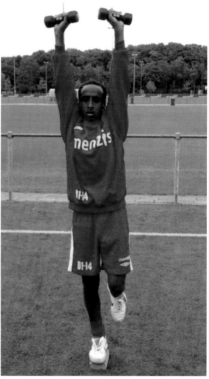

Photo 138e: Touch the weights to the ground again.

Photo 138f: Make a smooth transition back into the single-leg balance pose.

16.2.2 PARTNER STRENGTH AND BALANCE TRAINING

By now it can be considered an empirically proven fact that training exercises on unstable support surfaces result in increased muscle activity during a movement and, thus, a higher training effect (Anderson and Behm, 2005). The following partner exercises closely approximate this principle of every athletic movement: **perturbation.** The constant struggle for balance in the following pulling and pushing battles is very demanding on the central nervous system, which "fights" by all available means to perform the movement task. Just like in a soccer duel, direction, timing, and extent of the opposing interference are largely unknown.

EXERCISE 1

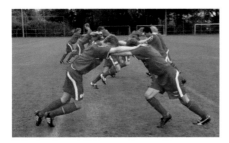 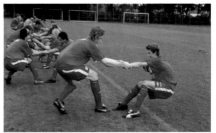

Photo 139a: Push your partner across the line.   *Photo 139b: Pull your partner across the line with a wrist-to-wrist grip.*

EXERCISE 2

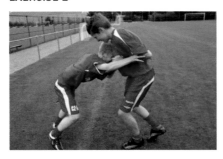 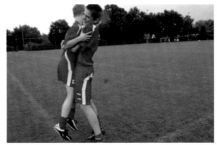

Photo 140a: Wrestling.   *Photo 140b: Try to lift each other off the ground.*

EXERCISE 3

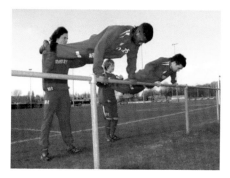 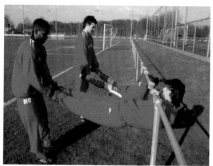

Photo 141a: Maintain body tension and perform push-ups with an overhand grip. The spotter uses a half-pinch grip.

Photo 141b: Perform pull-ups with an overhand grip in a horizontal position; the partner safeguards with a half-pinch grip so the player is able to maintain body tension.

EXERCISE 4

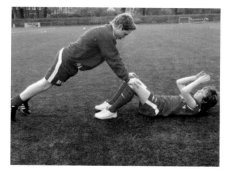 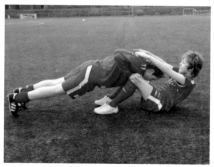

Photo 142a: One player performs push-ups against his partner's knees, using a half-pinch grip.

Photo 142b: The other player crunches up and touches his partner's back with his hands. Synchronized effort!

EXERCISE 5

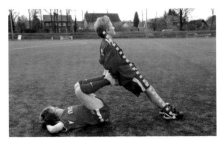 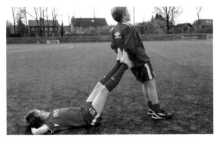

Photo 143a: Partner leg-press. Feet are parallel, pressing against the back in the sacral area. The partner's palms (in full body tension) are placed against the soles of the shoes. No cleats, please!

Photo 143b: The passive partner maintains body tension.

EXERCISE 6

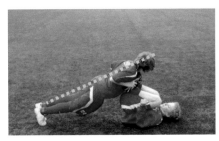 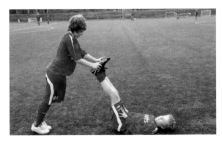

Photo 144a: Perform push-ups with a half-pinch grip.

Photo 144b: The partner performs a legpress.

EXERCISE 7

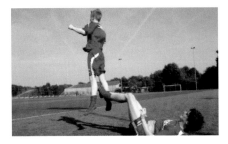 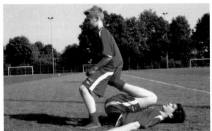

Photo 145a: Catapult: Keep your balance during the flight phase and land safely on both feet.

Photo 145b: Feet are placed against the partner's back. No cleats, please!

EXERCISE 8

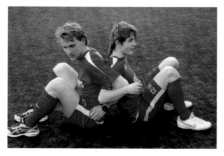 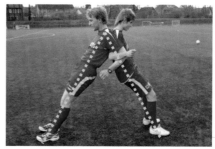

Photo 146a: Link arms and sit on the ground.   *Photo 146b: Coordinate standing up, keep your balance, and fully extend your body.*

EXERCISE 9

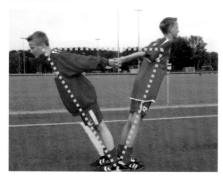

Photo 147: Vairplane with finger or wrist-to-wrist grip. Keep your balance!

EXERCISE 10

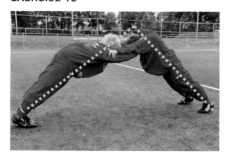

Photo 148: Airplane with half pinch grip. How far can you move apart without losing your balance?

EXERCISE 11: TUG-OF-WAR

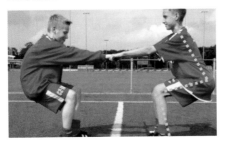 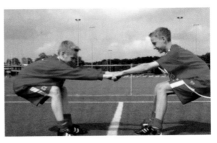

Photo 149a: Use a bar to maintain a 90-degree angle.

Photo 149b: The players must try to pull each other off position.

EXERCISE 12

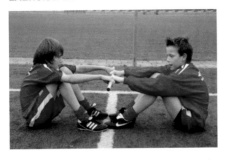 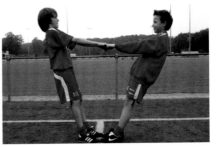

Photo 150a: Use an overhand grip on the pole.

Photo 150b: Standing up, keep arms and trunk extended.

EXERCISE 13

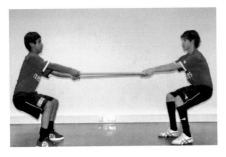 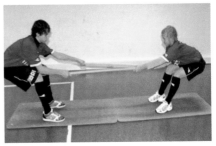

Photo 151a: Hold two poles at their ends with a half-pinch grip and bend your knees at a 90-degree angle.

Photo 151b: Try to pull the partner off balance. Who is the first to move his feet?

EXERCISE 14

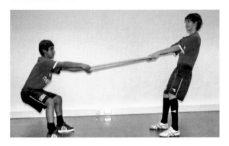 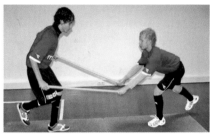

Photo 152a: See-saw: Take turns bending and straightening legs with arms extended and hands holding the ends of two poles in a half-pinch grip, maintaining balance.

Photo 152b: Balance on one leg! Competition: See who is the first to shift his supporting leg (-1 point) or has to use his second leg (-2 points). Regularly switch the supporting leg.

EXERCISE 15

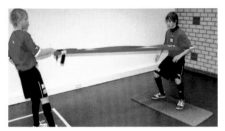 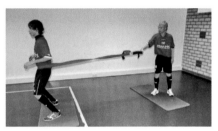

Photo 153a: Keep your balance against the pulling motions by means of the Reivo Elastic Band.

Photo 153b: One player cannot see the other. Tighten, relax!

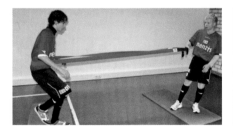 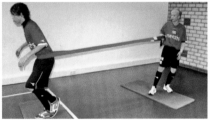

Photo 153c: The player standing on one leg tries to balance against suddenly decreasing or increasing tension of the Reivo Band without losing his balance.

Photo 153d: Same as photo c, but now with his back to his partner.

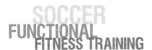
EXERCISE 16

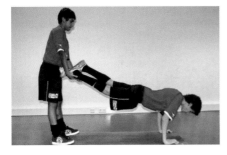 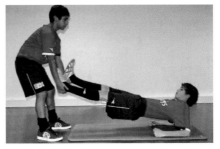

Photo 154a: The player tries to maintain the pictured push-up position with his partner's help. The partner releases his open grip (palm up) without warning (left or right).

Photo 154b: Here, the exercise is done in a reverse elbow plank position.

EXERCISE 17

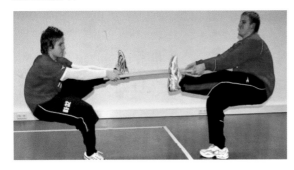

Photo 155: Kazachoc with two poles held in a half-pinch grip. Alternately touch the poles with the inside and outside foot.

EXERCISE 18

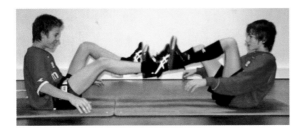

Photo 156: In a seated position with legs extended, bicycle together while maintaining trunk tension.

VARIATIONS:

1. Catching legs while in a seated balance: One partner quickly moves his closed legs up and down. The other partner tries to catch them by closing his legs around them while also in a seated balance.

2. Same as variation 1, but arms are crossed in front of the chest.
3. Leg pushing: See which partner falls over first or uses his arms for support. Hold competitions.

EXERCISE 19

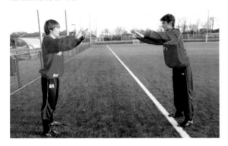 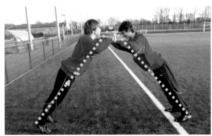

Photo 157a: Stand approximately body-length apart.

Photo 157b: Fall into each other's extended arms, withpalms interlocked to absorb the impact. After hand contact, firmly push off, extending the arms again. Players should return to the secure starting position. Caution: Maintain eye contact and agree in advance on a command to prevent head injuries.

EXERCISE 20

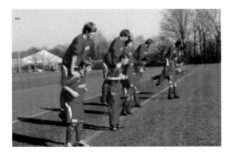

Photo 158: Jumping and bracing—the partner's shoulders provide the supporting surface.

EXERCISE 21

Photo 159: Climbing tree: One player tries to climb around his partner as quickly as possible without touching the ground. Hold competitions between pairs.

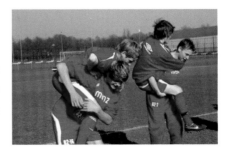

EXERCISE 22

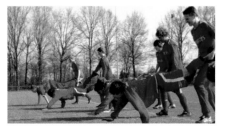

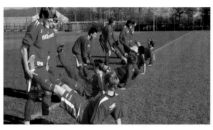

Photo 160a: Wheelbarrow in push-up position. The partner safeguards with an open grip (palms up).

Photo 160b: Variation: Wheelbarrow in reverse plank position. Hold competitions.

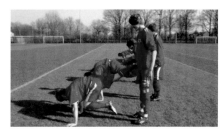

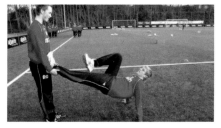

Photo 160c: In push-up position, alternately bring the free leg into the chest. The partner safeguards by always holding one leg with an open grip.

Photo 160d: The player must alternately pull one knee into the chest.

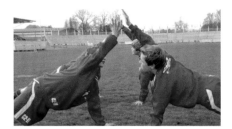

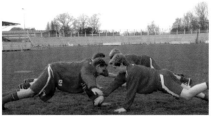

Photo 160e: From a push-up position, alternately bring your palms together. Stretch high and high-five!

Photo 160f: Maintain body tension! Who will be he first to lose his balance and drop to his stomach? Rule: Players are allowed to touch their partner's arms. Competition: See which player is the first to score three points.

VARIATION:

❯ Rock-paper-scissors: Both players simultaneously lift, for example, the right hand and on command perform these familiar hand signals. Hold competitions (push-up battle).

EXERCISE 23

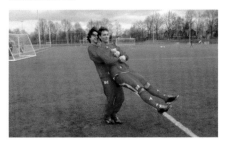

Photo 161: Carousel: Make the partner "fly" by gripping him around the chest or with another type of grip, and turning, take small steps.

EXERCISE 24

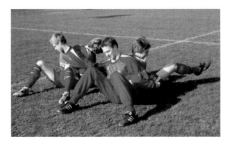

Photo 162: Try to push each other sideways to the ground! Sit back to back and link arms.

EXERCISE 25

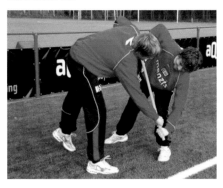

Photo 163: Try to push one end of the pole to the ground against the partner's resistance. Caution: Keep the upper end of the pole away from the partner's head!

EXERCISE 26

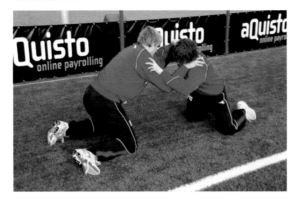

Photo 164: In a kneeling position and with hands on each other's shoulders, try to push the partner off balance and sideways to the ground.

EXERCISE 27

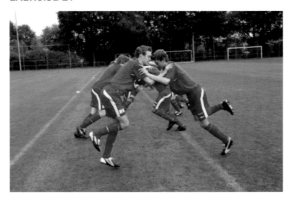

Photo 165: Hopping, pushing, and balancing on one leg: Who is the first to leave the marked lane or to touch the ground with the free leg?

EXERCISE 28

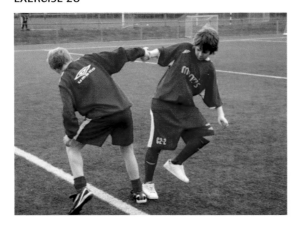

Photo 166: Balance on one leg and pull each other with a wrist-to-wrist grip: Which player is able to balance for 10 seconds?

EXERCISE 29

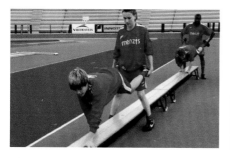 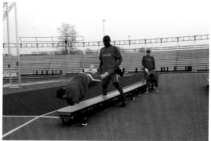

Photo 167a: Wheelbarrow on a long bench.

Photo 167b: Zigzag wheelbarrow over a long bench.

EXERCISE 30

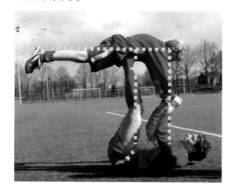

Photo 168: Forward-facing airplane: Keep your balance! Both feet (without shoes) rest against the rectus abdominis below the sternum. Caution: Please provide explicit advanced demonstration of foot placement and call attention to the players' great responsibility toward the "airplane." Prevent crashes!

EXERCISE 31

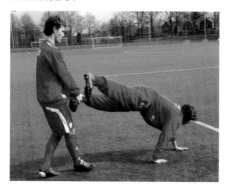

Photo 169: Wheelbarrow with one free leg. Competition: Five yards to the line, turn around while switching the free leg, and go back to the start. Hold competitions!

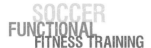
EXERCISE 32

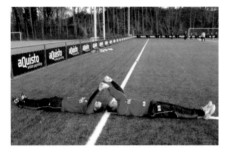 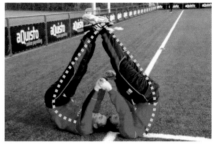

Photo 170a: In a supine position, lock hands with arms extended.

Photo 170b: Lift legs (resting on shoulders) and let your feet touch your partner's.

EXERCISE 33

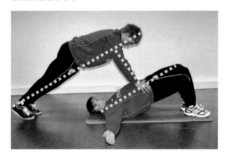

Photo 171: Push-up vs. bridge

EXERCISE 34

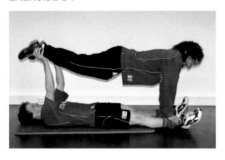

Photo 172: Synchronized extension and flexion using a pinch grip

EXERCISE 35

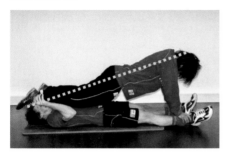

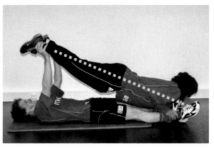

Photo 173a: Partners take turns straightening their arms.

Photo 173b: The partner without floor contact stabilizes his body like a board.

EXERCISE 36

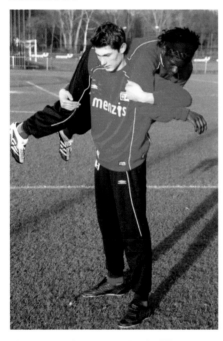

EXERCISE 37

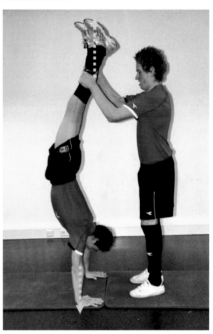

Photo 174: Take turns running in different ways while carrying the partner across the shoulders. For advanced athletes only.

Photo 175: Perform vertical push-ups with partner assistance.

EXERCISE 38

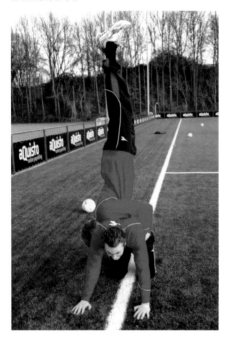

Photo 176: The player clasps his arms around his partner, who is in a stable table position. By extending his entire body, the player tries to get into a shoulder stand while balancing with his partner's help.

EXERCISE 39

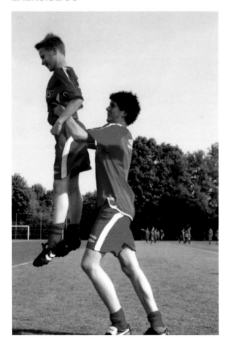

Photo 177: The player vigorously lifts his partner with a half-pinch grip and lets him "fly." This partner, in turn, gathers momentum on the ground (going down and up). Landing should be soft.

EXERCISE 40: ACROBATICS

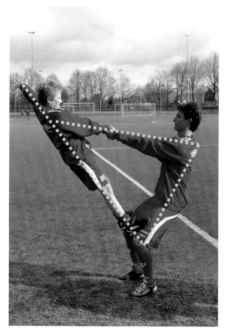

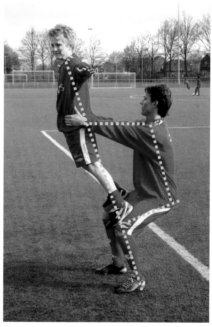

Photo 178a: Chair: Wrist-to-wrist grip and use indoor soccer or gym shoes. Variation: Both players hold one arm to the side.

Photo 178b: Figurehead: The partner securely holds the player in the pelvic area using a pinch grip.

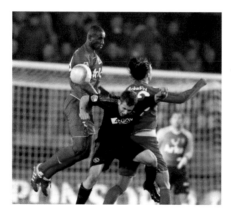

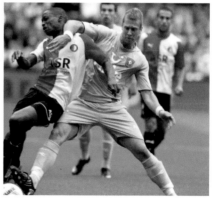

Photo 178c: Practical test in elite soccer—duels in the air with extreme risk.

Photo 178d: Physical contact and still keeping possession! Today's elite soccer.

EXERCISE 41

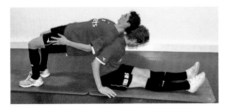

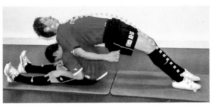

Photo 179a: Make a bridge against your partner's back.

Photo 179b: Flexibility is key.

EXERCISE 42

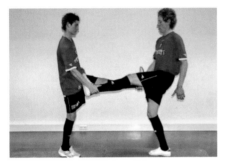

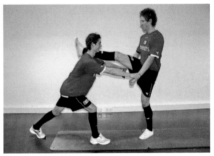

Photo 180a: Hopping in a circle on one leg, both players stabilize the motion sequence with half-pinch grips.

Photo 180b: The partner must now try to raise one leg without losing his balance. The leg should be raised carefully!

EXERCISE 43

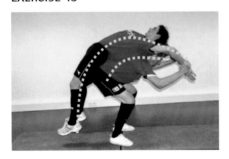

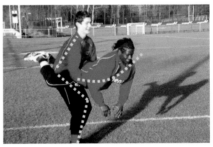

Photo 181a: Form two arches and keep your balance.

Photo 181b: Swing the partner left and right (controlled swing). The partner steadies himself and pushes off against the ground with his hands (elastic but with power).

EXERCISE 44

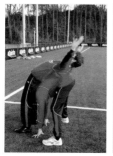 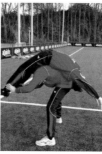 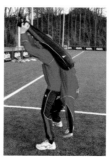 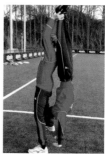

Photo 182, a-d: The partner stands in a secure straddle position while also steadying himself with his hands against the ground. The player stands in front of his partner in a straddle, facing away from him, and slowly bends over backwards with his arms extended, creating physical contact with his partner. He holds the player above the ankles with a half-pinch grip. By steadily and smoothly raising his upper body, the partner now lowers the player into a handstand. This exercise can be finished by reassuming the starting position orfinish the dismount with a handstand (advanced skills). The pictured reversal can also be performed as a separate exercise. Here the player starts out by performing a handstand against the back of his upright partner. He holds on to the player's calves with a half-pinch grip, lowers his upper body, and pulls the player forward and down in a smooth and controlled motion.

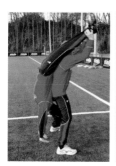 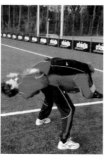 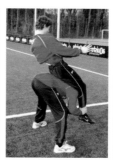 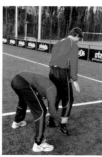

Photo 182, e-h: Reversing to the starting position (see photo 182, a-d). It is recommended to begin with exercise 44 (and its variation) with four players. The two additional players are performing the previously mentioned hand support to stabilize the player's center. This helps to keep the legs from flipping over too quickly or the arms from buckling during the support phase.

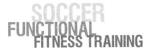
16.2.3 THREE-MAN STRENGTH AND BALANCE TRAINING

Assisting each other, training in groups, and maintaining a high level of motivation and the willingness to try hard is increasingly more important to coaches and instructors in today's soccer.

> *Cooperating, competing,* and *communicating* are educational aspects of responsible, performance-oriented soccer training. The team, social, action, and decision-making competences that evolve from this do not fall into one's lap and should be initiated didactically and methodically every day by the coach or /instructor, particularly during individually performed athletic training.*

The following exercises pertain to this and will integrate particularly the joyful world of experience for performance-oriented youth players into strength and athletic training withgroups of three. Mindless athletic training should be a thing of the past.

EXERCISE 1

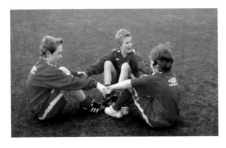

Photo 183a: Sit toe to toe in a group of three.

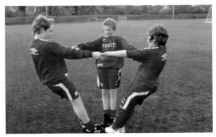

Photo 183b: Use subsequent leg extension. Total-body extension and firm grip!

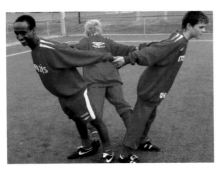

Photo 183c: Players are back to back and try to maintain their balance.

EXERCISE 2

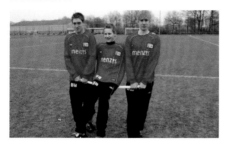 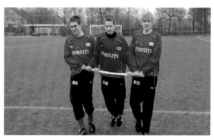

Photo 184a: See chapter 15.The player being carried must balance by himself during the prearranged relay game.

Photo 184b: The middle player is now in a push-up position using an overhand grip and tries to maintain his balance without touching the ground during a relay race.

EXERCISE 3

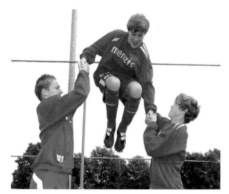

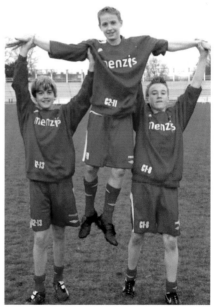

Photo 185a: Two players support the third player with support grips during a vertical jump. Go into a tuck at the highest point!

VARIATIONS:

- ❂ Tuck and turn.
- ❂ Two hip-high basic jumps are combined with a maximum height basic jump with partner assistance. Create sequences!
- ❂ Turn during the jump (forward-backwards-left-right).

Photo 185b: The partners support and carry the player for several yards using half-pinch grips, as shown. Form relay teams and hold competitions.

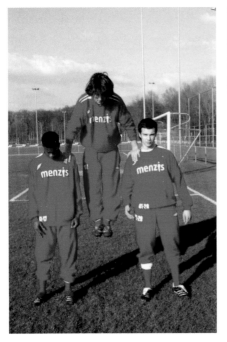

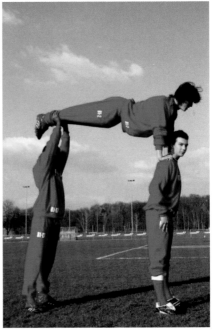

Photo 185c: The middle player jumps up from a standing position and braces himself against his partners' shoulders (supported jump). Due to risk of injury, the partners are not allowed to move to the side. Holdthe support position for approximately 3 seconds.

Photo 185d: Airplane: In the pictured version, participants walk together for approximately 10 yards. Caution: Try first in a kneeling position and assess the players' strength abilities. Possibly add more players for additional safeguarding support.

EXERCISE 4

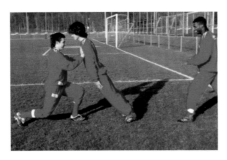

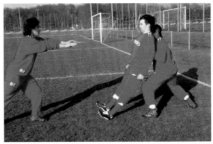

Photo 186a: Trust and body tension.

Photo 186b: Catching softly in a lunge position.

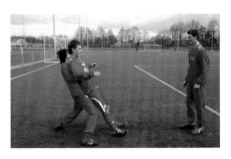

Photo 186c: Push the upright and rigid player (board) back and forth.

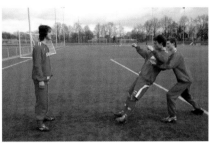

Photo 186d: The inside player continually turns 180 degrees. The teammates should decelerate the body early. Cooperation is key!

EXERCISE 5

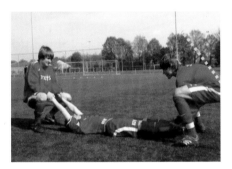

Photo 187a: Pulling motions and body tension. Don't pull with your back!

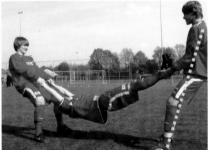

Photo 187b: By straightening their legs and shifting the long axes of their bodies into opposite directions, the partners pull the player from a squat into a horizontal position. Then they gradually unload and carefully lower the player to the ground. Backs should remain as straight as possible (see dotted line).

EXERCISE 6

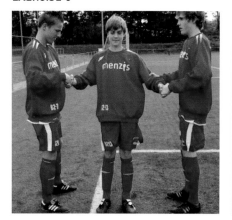

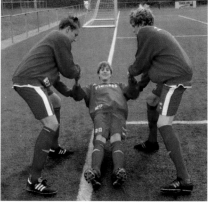

Photo 188a: Dead man: The partners hold on to the player with a half-pinch and wrist-to-wrist grip.

Photo 188b: The partners cushion the backwards falling motion with a side lunge. Once the player is in a stable horizontal position, he is held there for approximately 3 seconds and then pulled back up into an upright position, while maintaining body tension.

EXERCISE 7

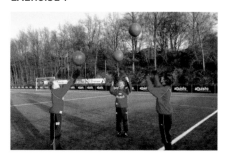

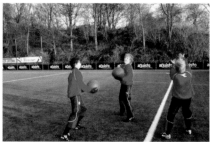

Photo 189a: The players toss the medicine balls into the air in sync with a push throw.

Photo 189b: After 12 throws, the players switch places clockwise or counterclockwise while the balls are in the air. The captain gives the signal. Players should stay in triangle formation. Communication trumps!

16.2.4 INDIVIDUAL ATHLETIC TRAINING WITH AN "ALL-ROUNDER" MEDICINE BALL

The medicine ball wasa proven piece of exercise equipment long before the media covered the fitness training of our very successful soccer instructor colleague Felix Magath. Moreover, it is part of the basic equipment of many fitness facilities and allows the coach and instructor to implement many training goals, such as coordination, sensorimotor skills, and fitness. From a fitness standpoint, the added weight of the medicine ball makes it possible to increase strength demands and initiate the power supply over time.

If the focus of training is to deflect familiar movements or make them more complex and to steady partial movements with the medicine ball in order to achieve training effects in other parts of the body, this tool facilitates top-notch coordination training. Furthermore, it is an additional methodological tool that provides the coach and instructor extensive organizational flexibility (stations, circuits, or laps and individual and group work), which ensures (individual) targeted load and demand metering and benefits emotional competence. Specifically, medicine balls with lots of tempo, large amounts of movement for players, and that use multiple balls simultaneously and are lots of fun.

The balls should be chosen deliberately. Balls that are too heavy or too old are a no-go, particularly in youth training. Developmentally appropriate plastic or rubber balls are generally the best choice on the practice field.

Safety measures should be scrutinized during training planning. Spatial arrangement of exercises on the soccer field should help prevent balls from rolling and flying at spectators, prevent players from stepping on them and rolling an ankle, and avoid safety distances that are too small (e.g., shocking and winding up).

A consistent warning and stop signal has proven beneficial in practice. Dangerous situations can,therefore, be recognized early and managed responsibly by all participants. The direct participation of players in this safety measure promotes good judgment.

Thus, the reputation of medicine ball athletic training as being antiquated fitness training is completely unjustified.

SOCCER
FUNCTIONAL
FITNESS TRAINING

EXERCISE 1

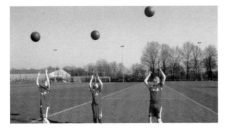

Photo 190a: Throw and push the ball into the air and catch it sitting down.

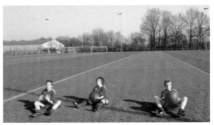

Photo 190b: Reversed execution: Throw the ball while sitting down; catch it standing up.

EXERCISE 2

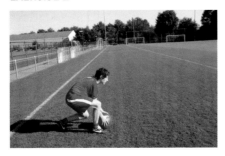

Photo 191a: Jump up from a lunge position, and alternate legs.

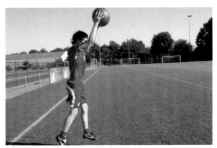

Photo 191b: Complete the jump from a lunge position with total-body extension.

EXERCISE 3

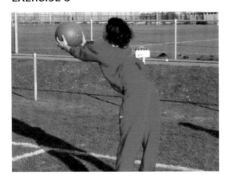

Photo 192a: In a standing position, first hold the medicine ball with arms extended forward, then throw it backwards in an overheadarc.

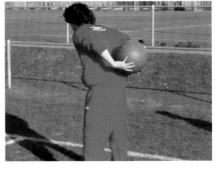

Photo 192b: Catch the medicine ball with both hands and without looking. Timing is everything, and try to stay as upright as possible!

EXERCISE 4

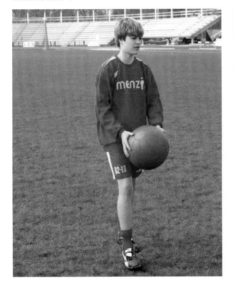 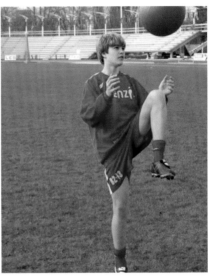

Photo 193a: Rest the medicine ball on one thigh and try to propel it into the air with a vigorous knee lift.

Photo 193b: Maintain total-body extension over the forward foot.

EXERCISE 5

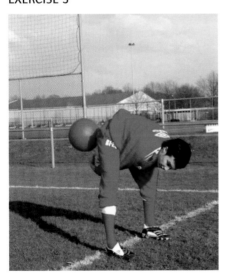 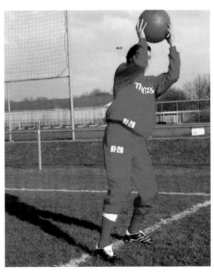

Photo 194a: Throw the ball back and up— through the legs and over the back to the front.

Photo 194b: Safely catch the ball.

EXERCISE 6

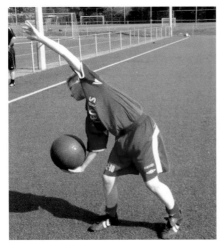

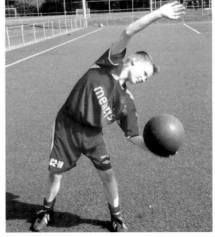

Photo 195a: Single-arm throws.

Photo 195b: Always bend the trunk firmly to the side.

EXERCISE 7

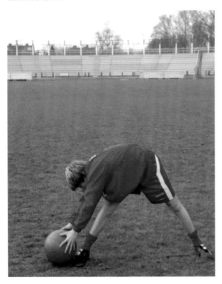

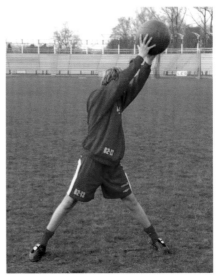

Photo 196a: In a straddle position, move the ball down and to the side.

Photo 196b: Then move the ball to the other side after doing a total-body extension. Try not to bend the knees.

EXERCISE 8

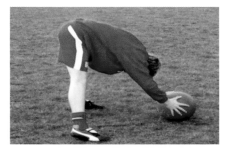

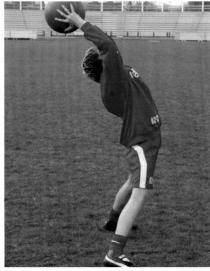

Photo 197a: Rest the medicine ball on the ground,as pictured, at a distance from your feet.

Photo 197b: Return to an upright position with the arms extended.

EXERCISE 9

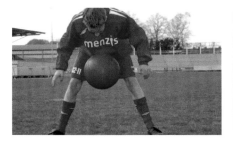

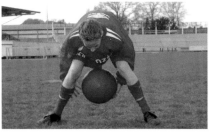

Photo 198a: Let go of the medicine ball, as pictured.

Photo 198b: Alternate catching the ball in front of and behind the legs with both hands.

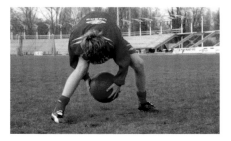

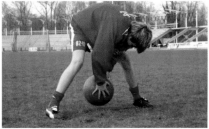

Photo 198c: Now catch the medicine ball on a diagonal.

Photo 198d: Twist the trunk after each catch.

EXERCISE 10

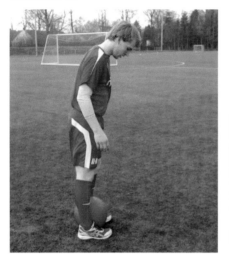

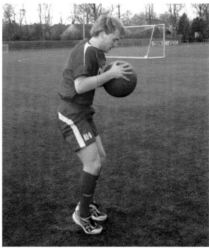

Photo 199a: Hold the medicine ball between your feet.

Photo 199b: Propel the medicine ball into the air with a jump, and then catch it.

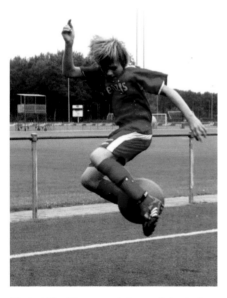

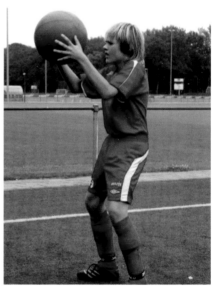

Photo 199c: Then propel the medicine ball up and forward with a sideways jump.

Photo 199d: Catch the ball as high as possible in front of the body.

EXERCISE 11

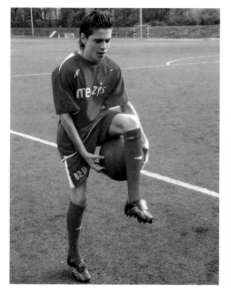

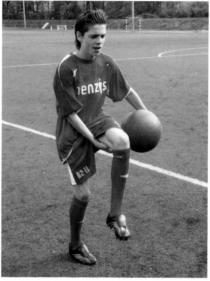

Photo 200a: Constantly alternate passing the ball from the inside to the outside at a lope.

Photo 200b: Pass the medicine ball to the inside from the outside of the knees.

EXERCISE 12

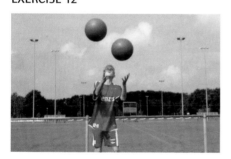

Photo 201: Juggle two medicine balls.

EXERCISE 13

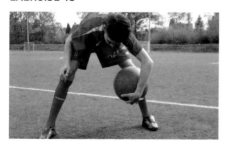

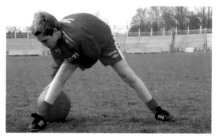

Photo 202a: Figure-eights between the legs.

Photo 202b: Roll the ball in figure-eights.

EXERCISE 14

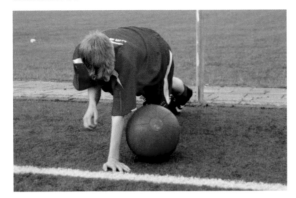

Photo 203: In a single-arm push-up, move the ball around the supporting arm.

EXERCISE 15

Photo 204a: Stand on one leg with the supporting foot on a wooden wedge or balance pad. Start by holding the medicine ball on the ground.

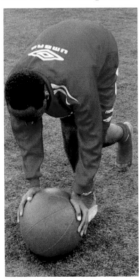

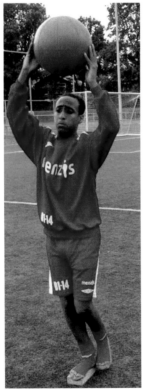

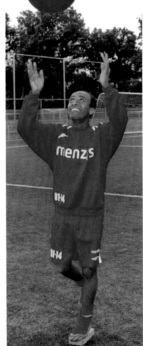

Photo 204b: Lift the medicine ball into a total-body extension while balancing.

Photo 204c: Variation: Toss the medicine ball into the air.

EXERCISE 16

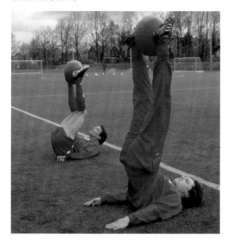

Photo 205: Move into a shoulder stand from a seated position with legs extended.

EXERCISE 17

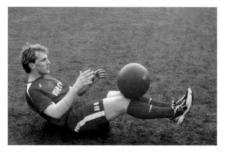

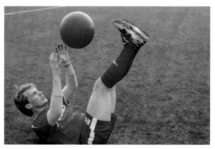

Photo 206a: Roll the medicine ball toward your feet while balancing.

Photo 206b: Bat the medicine ball forward and upward with your legs, and then catch it with your hands while raising your trunk.

EXERCISE 18

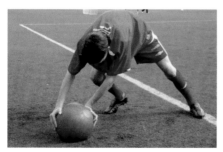

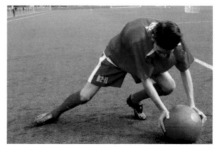

Photo 207a: Jump side to side while bracing against the medicine ball.

Photo 207b: Make sure that the outside leg is extended as much as possible.

EXERCISE 19

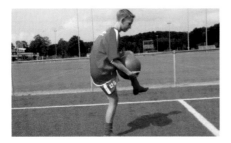

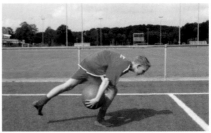

Photo 208a: Stand on one leg and raise the other leg. Don't wearshoes.

Photo 208b: Extend the raised leg back and then pass the medicine ball between legs (as pictured). Keep your balance! Variation: Choose different support surfaces.

EXERCISE 20

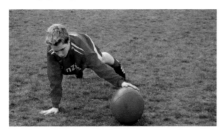

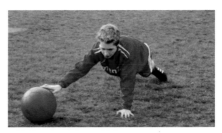

Photo 209a: Roll the medicine ball side to side in a push-up position.

Photo 209b: Roll the medicine ball farther away from the body.

EXERCISE 21: WITH HANDS ON THE BALL

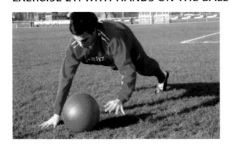

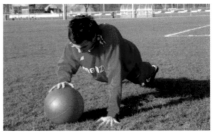

Photo 210a: In push-up position, alternate the supporting hand on the ball with a little jump.

Photo 210b: Make sure the elbows are bent.

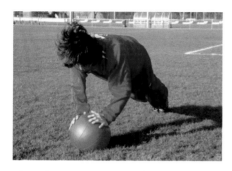 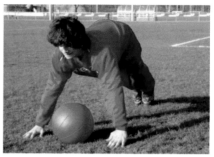

Photo 210c: Support yourself with both hands on the medicine ball.

Photo 210d: Vigorously push off the medicine ball andsoftly land on the ground (bend-extend-bend-extend). Variation: Explosive push-ups in which the ball briefly loses contact with the ground after the extension phase.

EXERCISE 22

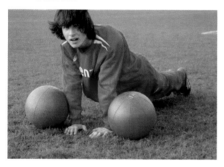 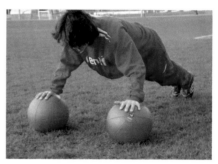

Photo 211a: See exercise 21. This exercise is very demanding on the players' strength abilities.

Photo 211b: Again, arms are not extended during the supporting phase.

EXERCISE 23

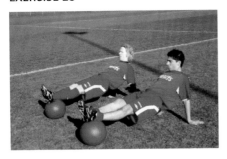

Photo 212a: Reverse plank with feet on the medicine ball. Hold for approximately 5 seconds.

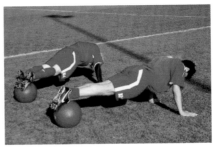

Photo 212b: Get into push-up position with feet on the medicine ball. Hold for approximately 5 seconds.

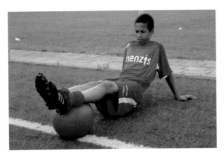

Photo 212c: Lift hips off the ground from a seated position.

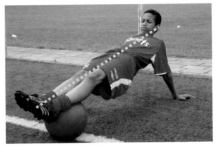

Photo 212d: Roll forward along the calves until the body is fully extended, followed by a reverse plank.

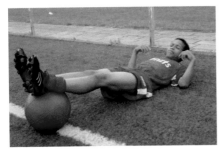

Photo 212e: Lift the hips off the ground from a supine position.

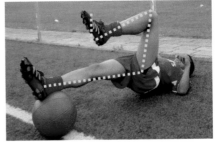

Photo 212d: Alternate lifting one knee, as pictured.Maintain hip extension and stable body position for approximately 3 seconds.

EXERCISE 24

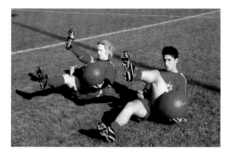

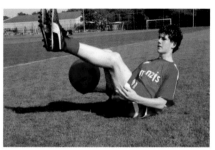

Photo 213a: Move legs in a scissors motion while passing the medicine ball between the legs, as pictured.

Photo 213b: Continuously pass the medicine ball around your nearly extended legs.

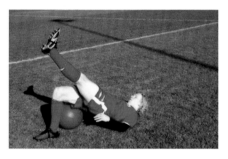

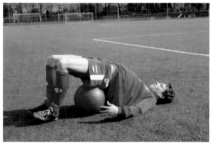

Photo 213c: Alternate legs in single-leg bridge position while rolling the medicine ball from side to side under the supporting leg.

Photo 213d: Get into bridge position with legs closed and roll the medicine side to side under your legs.

EXERCISE 25

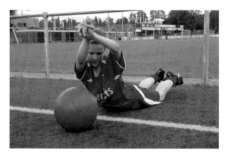

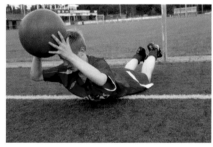

Photo 214a: Rock back and forth with arms extended over the medicine ball.

Photo 214b: Rock back and forth while holding the medicine ball with arms extended.

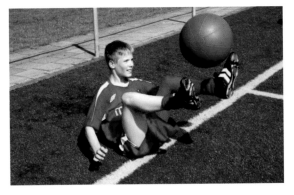

EXERCISE 26

Photo 215: In a seated position, toss the medicine ball into the air and catch it using your feet. The trunk should remain as straight as possible.

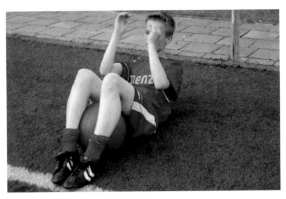

EXERCISE 27

Photo 216: Clamp the medicine ball, as pictured, while performing crunches.

EXERCISE 28

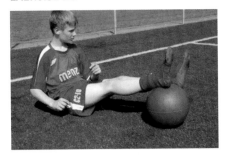 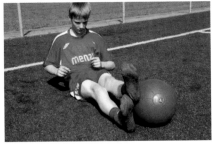

Photo 217a: Put pressure on the medicine ball: Keeping your legs closed, press down on the medicine ball, alternating legs while balancing.

Photo 217b: Keep the trunk as straight as possible.

EXERCISE 29

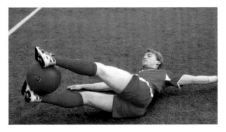 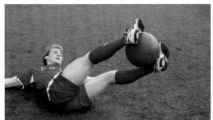

Photo 218a: Windshieldwiper: Position the legs as straight as possible at a 90-degree angle.

Photo 218b: Do not let your legs touch the ground. Keep arms in Tposition help with balance. Keep your shoulders on the ground!

EXERCISE 30

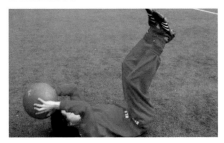 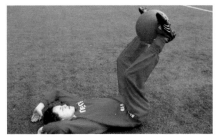

Photo 219a: Hand-off: The medicine ball is now sandwiched between the feet.

Photo 219b: The movement is reversed. Keep legs as straight as possible.

EXERCISE 31

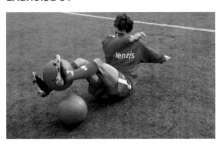 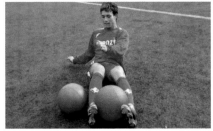

Photo 220a: Seated windshieldwiper: Pay particular attention to the countermovement of the arms.

Photo 220b: Move the extended legs from one side of the medicine ball to the other without setting them down on the medicine ball.

EXERCISE 32

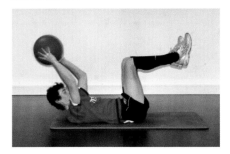

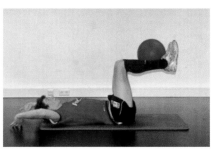

Photo 221a: Ball transfer: Continuously alternate transferring the medicine ball to the bent legs.

Photo 221b: The medicine ball is held between the shins, and the trunk is in supine position.

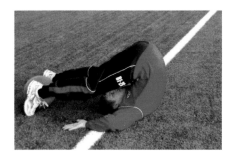

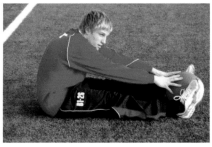

Photo 221c: From a seated position with legs extended, move legs into a plow position with the medicine ball between the feet, and let the feet briefly touch the ground.

Photo 221d: After rolling back into a seated position, touch the ball with the hands.

EXERCISE 33

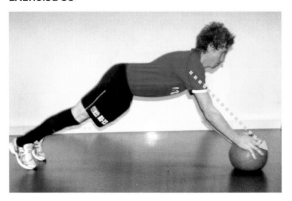

Photo 222: In a push-up position, roll the medicine ball as far forward as possible and then back again.

EXERCISE 34

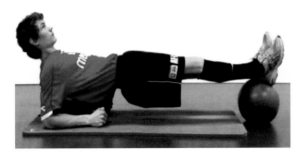

Photo 223: Reverse forearm plank: Lift and lower hips and hold for approximately 3 seconds.

EXERCISE 35

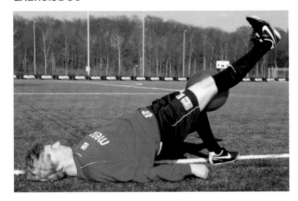

Photo 224: Single-leg bridge with medicine ball, alternating legs.

EXERCISE 36

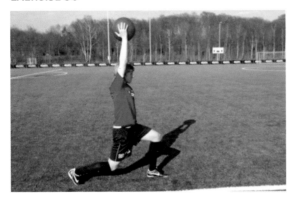

Photo 225a: Lunges: Controlled forward and back lunges with the ball held high overhead. Focus on body tension with an upright trunk andlegalignment, and avoid an acute angle of the knee.

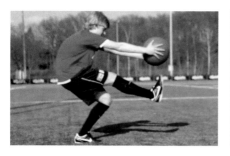

Photo 225b: The player holds the medicine ball with his arms extended forward and does alternating single-leg squats. Keep balance.

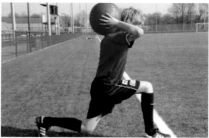

Photo 225c: Lunge from a standing position with the medicine ball held behind the head. Variation: Hold the ball to the chest.The forward knee must not come out over the toe. The extended leg touches the medicine ball. Next switch the supporting leg, and repeat.

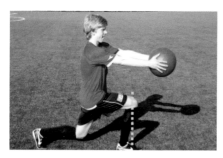

Photo 225d: Lunge while holding the medicine ball with arms extended in front of the body. The knee never comes out over the toe.

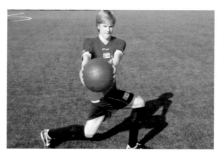

Photo 225e: Add 90-degree trunk rotations and forward and back lunges.

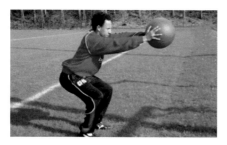

Photo 225f: Do a half squat with parallel feet. Knee angles can be modified.

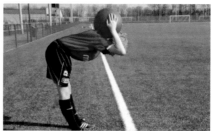

Photo 225g: Good mornings: Be careful not to hyperextend the knees.

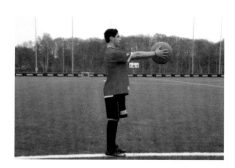

Photo 225h: Get into the starting position for warrior IIIpose.

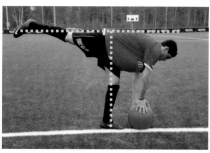

Photo 225i: Transition to warrior III (notice the visible longitudinal and sagittal axes).

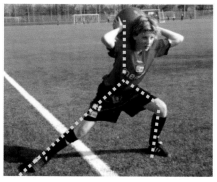

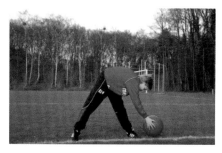

Photo 225k: Initiate a low to high motion with the medicine ball.

Photo 225j: Alternate side lunges. Keep the trunk up with the medicine ball behind the head.

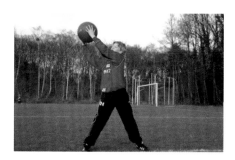

Photo 225l: Complete the diagonal movement. Switch sides. It can also be performed as a three-dimensional variation.

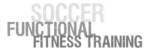

EXERCISE 37

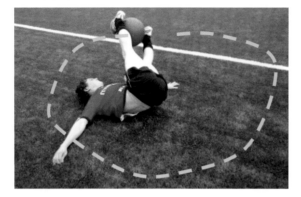

Photo 226: Protractor: Move your legs in a circle withthe medicine ball between your lower legs. Reverse directions.

EXERCISE 38

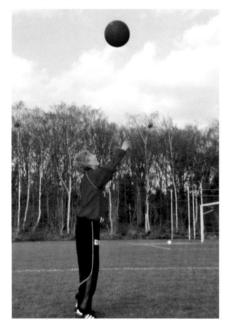

EXERCISE 39

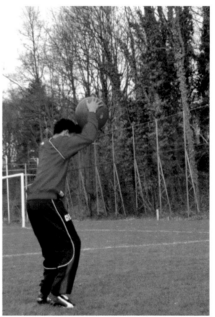

Photo 227: Holding the medicine ball with arms extended forward in a half squat, toss the ball into the air and then catch it.

Photo 228: From a total-body extension, bounce the medicine ball on the ground and then catch it.

EXERCISE 40

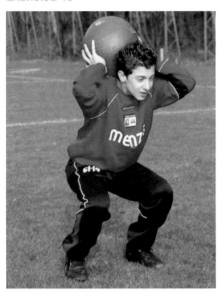

Photo 229a: Toss the medicine ball up from a half squat.

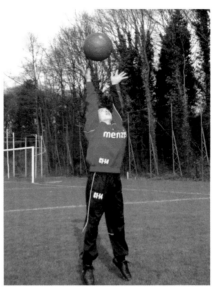

Photo 229b: Maintain the subsequent dynamic total-body extension.

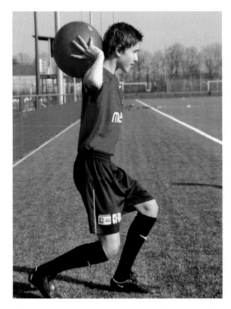

Photo 229c: From a lunge position, toss the medicine ball as high as possible into the air.

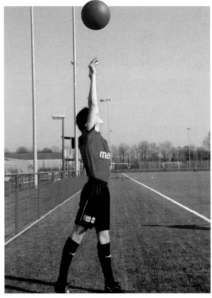

Photo 229d: At the same time, perform a total-body extension.

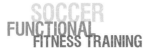

16.2.5 PARTNER ATHLETIC TRAINING WITH AN "ALL-ROUNDER" MEDICINE BALL

EXERCISE 1

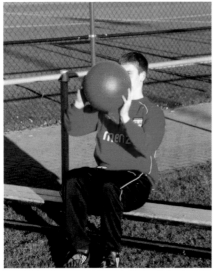 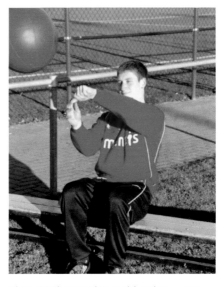

Photo 230a: Throw the ball from a seated position, using both arms. One player throws; the other playercatches and throws back.

Photo 230b: Now throw with only one arm.

EXERCISE 2

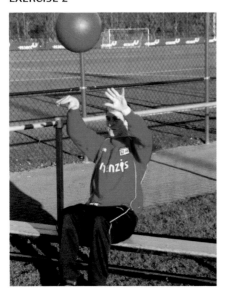

Photo 231: Perform a throw-in from a seated position.

EXERCISE 3

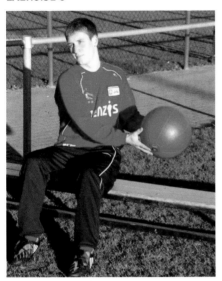

Photo 232: Throw from the side using both arms. Alternate sides.

EXERCISE 4

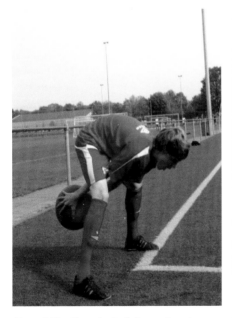

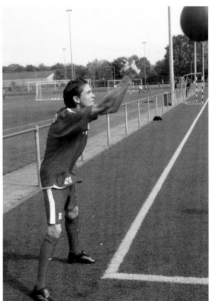

Photo 233a: Toss the ball forward and up, as pictured.

Photo 233b: Keep total-body extension up on the toes. The momentum originates in the legs.

EXERCISE 5

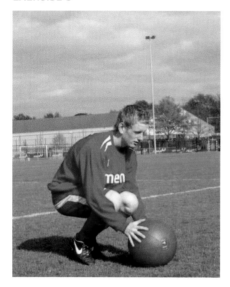

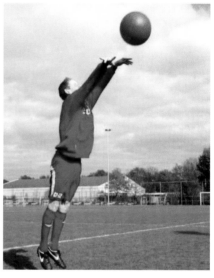

Photo 234a: Make a powerful throw from a squat position.

Photo 234b: Palms follow through. Throw high and far!

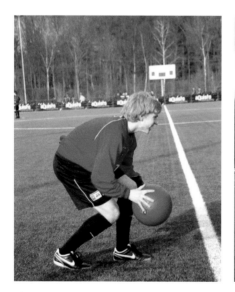

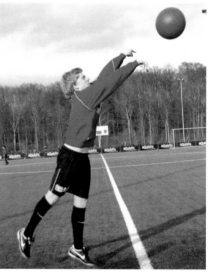

Photo 234c: Explosively throw the medicine ball while moving from a squat into a lunge position.

Photo 234d: Add a subsequent jumping motion accompanied by total-body extension.

EXERCISE 6

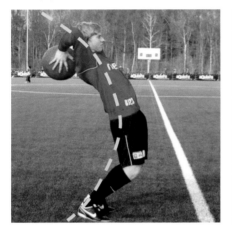 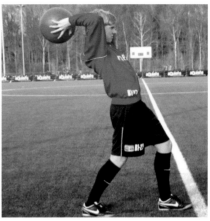

Photo 235a: Perform a throw-in with a closed stance. Bend the bow!

Photo 235b: Now throw in lunge position.

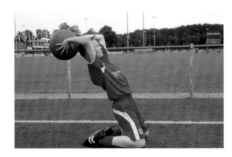 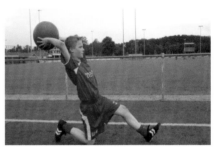

Photo 235c: Perform a kneeling throw-in.

Photo 235d: Perform throw-in on one knee with a bracing step.

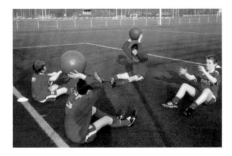 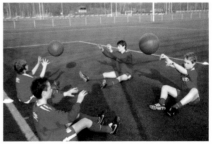

Photo 235e: Perform a seated throw-in.

Photo 235f: Perform a seated ball toss.

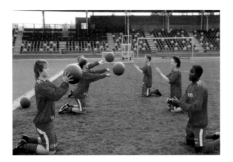

Photo 235g: Perform a kneeling ball toss as a group.

EXERCISE 7

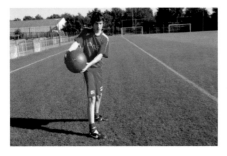

Photo 236a: Perform side throws with rotation in lunge position.

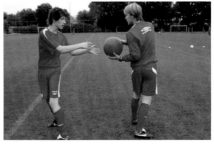

Photo 236b: Rollercoaster: Partners stand back to back at a distance of approximately two arm lengths. In a straddle position, both partners simultaneously twist in the same direction. One player passes the ball to the other player.

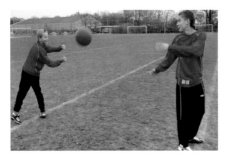

Photo 236c: The distance between players increases, and the medicine ball is thrown sideways with precision.

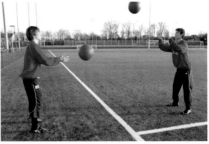

Photo 236d: Cabaret: Two players face each other, each with a medicine ball. They simultaneously toss each other a ball without the balls touching in the air.

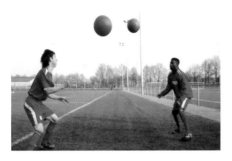

Photo 236e: Simultaneously throw both medicine balls from an offset position.

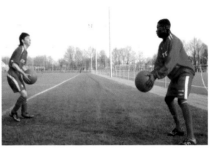

Photo 236f: Chase and catch the medicine balls in a side shuffle. One player sets the rhythm.

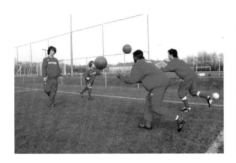

Photo 236g: Toss the medicine ball back and forth while standing on one leg. Keep balance!

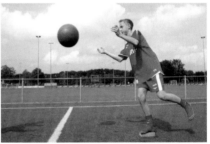

Photo 236h: Now balance on a wooden wedge or balance pad while tossing the ball back and forth.

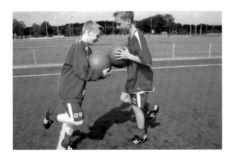

Photo 237a: Ball pressure: Players must try to push each other off balance with the medicine balls.

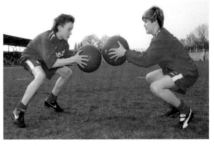

Photo 237b: The players must now try to push each other off balance in a squat position.

EXERCISE 9

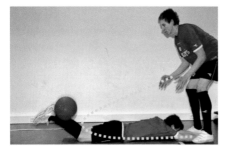 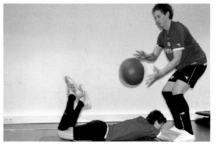

Photo 238a: The partner rolls the medicine ball along the back of the player lying on the floor.

Photo 238b: The player tries to accelerate the return ball to his partner by using his calves. Is the partner able to catch the ball?

EXERCISE 10

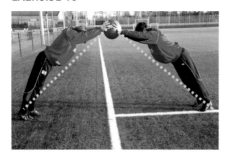

Photo 239a: Push-up wobble: Leaning toward each other with good traction, players wedge the ball between them with arms fully extended. This requires whole-body muscle tension and making sure the posterior does not push out too far. Body control is more important here than being the maximum distance apart.

VARIATIONS:

1. Start by performing push-ups close to the body.
2. In the final position, together transport the ball by taking small side steps.
3. Like variation 2, but with a marked course: parallel lines, triangles, or diamonds.
4. Pass the medicine ball in a row using several partner pairs.

VARIATION:

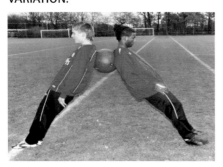

❂ In a back-to-back squat, transport the ball.

Photo 239b: Back-to-back action.

EXERCISE 11

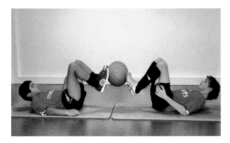 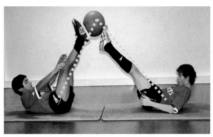

Photo 240a: Together support the medicine ball with the feet.

Photo 240b: Support the medicine ball with a leg extension. Maintain body tension, particularly on the ventral side, and put pressure against the ball.

EXERCISE 12

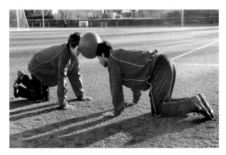 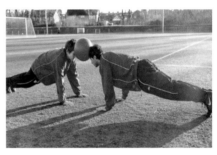

Photo 241a: Header duel: Put pressure against the ball in a kneeling position.

Photo 241b: Transition to a push-up.

EXERCISE 13

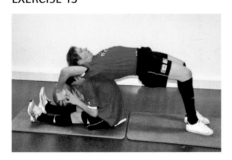 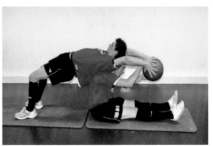

Photo 242a: Build a bridge and pass the ball underneath the bridge.

Photo 242b: Alternate. Maintain muscle tension!

EXERCISE 14

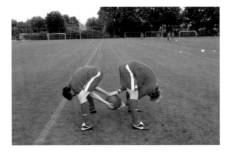 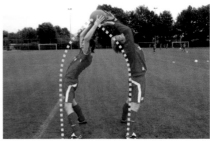

Photo 243a: Lumberjack: In a slight straddle position, bend over and pass the medicine ball through the legs.

Photo 243b: Move into an upright position and pass the ball overhead. Track the ball with your eyes.

EXERCISE 15

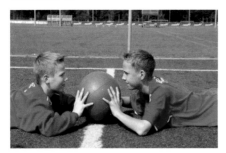 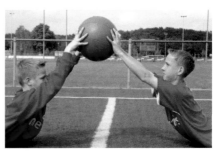

Photo 244a: Pressure on the ball: Steady the medicine ball in prone position with elbows bent.

Photo 244b: Together push the medicine ball upward. Stretch! Then gradually lower back down.

EXERCISE 16

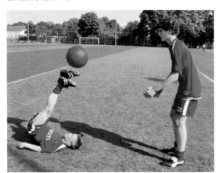

Photo 245: Foot catapult: Lying on your back, wedge the medicine ball between the legs and catapult it to the partner.

EXERCISE 17

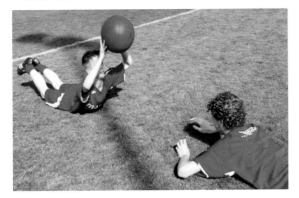

Photo 246: Belly see-saw: From a prone position, throw the medicine ball to the partner, steady and high.

EXERCISE 18

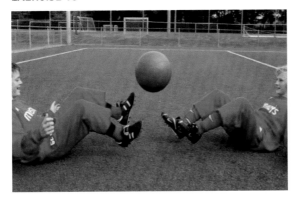

Photo 247: Seated double-leg juggling: Continuously catch the medicine ball with both legs.Return it to thepartner with a controlled toss using the legs.

EXERCISE 19

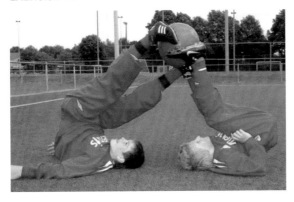

Photo 248: From a seated position with legs extended, roll back and pass the ball to the partner with your feet.

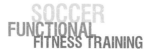
EXERCISE 20

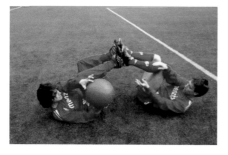 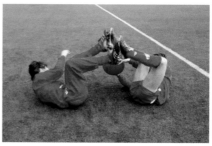

Photo 249a: Pattex: Continuously move the medicine ball around the legs and hand it off at the side.

Photo 249b: Maintain constant foot contact.

EXERCISE 21

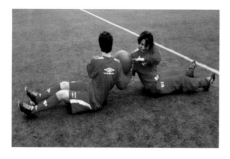 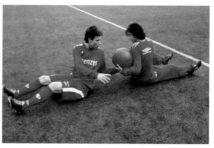

Photo 250a: Seated rollercoaster: In a seated position with legs extended, pass and receive the ball.

Photo 250b: Choose the distance so the partners can turn with the medicine ball without touching.

EXERCISE 22

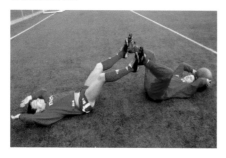

Photo 251: Pass the medicine ball in a supine position with legs raised and feet touching (Pattex) by rolling up and tossing the ball.

EXERCISE 23

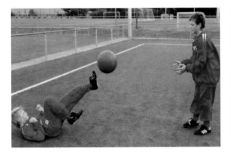

Photo 252a: One partner pushes the thrown medicine ball back to the other partner with the bottomof one foot.

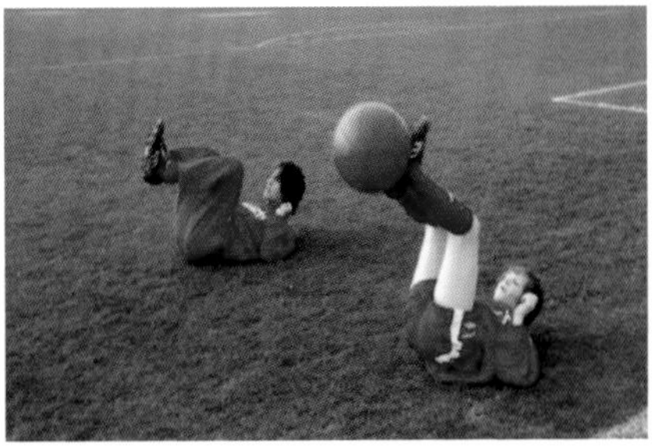

Photo 252b: Push the ball back to the partner with both feet.

EXERCISE 24

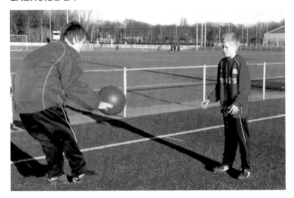

Photo 253: Flicking: In a standing position, wedge the medicine ball between your feet, jump up, and throw the ball to your partner. If possible the partner should catch the medicine ball with both feet.

EXERCISE 25

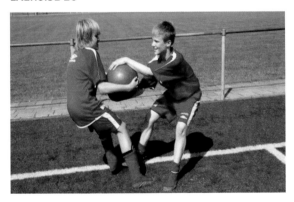

Photo 254: Ball wrestling: Which player is able to capture the ball?

EXERCISE 26

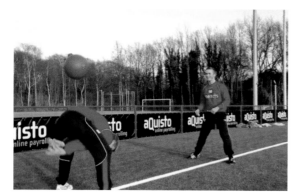

Photo 255: Toss the ball forward from behind.

EXERCISE 27

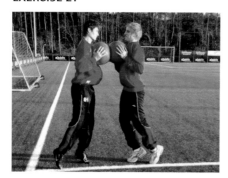

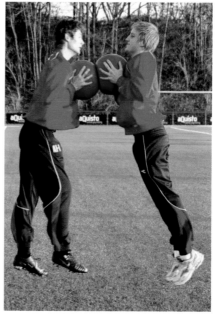

Photo 256a: Crash: Move toward each other with medicine balls held to the chest, and bump into each other. Hand position should be as shown.

Photo 256b: Now bump into each other with a jump. Make sure actions are simultaneous!

EXERCISE 28

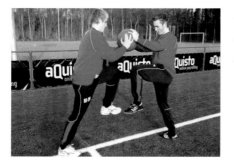

Photo 257: Knee lift with medicine ball: Stay in the depicted position for approximately 3 seconds and keep your balance!

EXERCISE 29

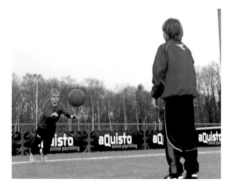

Photo 258: Frog: From a squat position, forcefully thrust the medicine ball at your partner. Follow through by landing on your stomach and rolling to the side.

VARIATIONS:

- Forward roll on a gymnastics mat.
- Judo roll.

EXERCISE 30

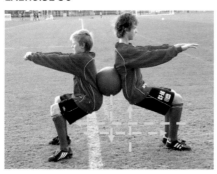

Photo 259: Shunting: Together, transport the ball in all directions with small steps.

VARIATION:

- Turns.

16.2.6 INDIVIDUAL ATHLETIC TRAINING WITH A KETTLEBELL

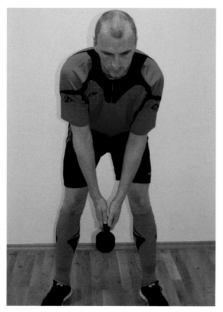

A kettlebell is a round weight with a U-shaped handle. Due to its special shape the kettlebell's center of gravity is not located in the center of the handle, but below the handle and, thus, outside the hand. In athletic training, this peculiarity gives the coach or instructor the option of working with curvilinear motions with rotations and centrifugal force. This type of varied loading and strain results in additional adaptations.

While most exercise equipment enables single- or double-joint movements, the kettlebell facilitates multi joint movements that are multi planar and close to whole-body movements. Consequently, forces affect the player on several planes and facilitate *heterolateral* and *homolateral* methods of training. The result is that muscles must perform more stabilizing work and, moreover, the cardiopulmonary load can be systematically controlled.

Furthermore, working with the kettlebell activates technical-coordinated abilities and skills and trains them. This is done primarily through swinging motions with the kettlebell that activate centrifugal force, as previously mentioned. The player is required to perform compensating motions to maintain his balance. This approximates today's soccer, where duels with quick turns (also without ground contact), quick twists and turns while dribbling, and falling with and without the ball have become regular key elements of modern competitive play.

Thus, kettlebell training presents an additional, versatile alternative for the development of all-around athletic soccer fitness.

As withstrength training in general, kettlebell training should be preceded by technique training with low weights that includes the following safety measures:

- Make sure that no one is in the training area.
- Secure one's training area by using gym mats and choosing kettlebells with a rubber coating.
- The weight is not lifted with the shoulders or arm strength, but from the corresponding leg movements and the lower trunk. The authors, therefore, recommend taking a beginner class and at this point refer to the fitness coach Paul Collins, who has written extensive documentation on the subject of kettlebells (2010).

Hereafter, the authors present practical training exercises that can be integrated into soccer athletic training.

EXERCISE 1: SINGLE- AND DOUBLE-ARM KETTLEBELL SWING

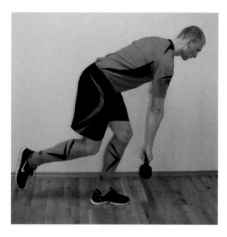

Starting position:

Keep knees slightly bent and make sure that the knee doesn't jut out over the toes of the supporting foot. Hold the kettlebell as shown in photo 260a, and do not round the back. The free arm compensates, maintaining balance.

Photo 260a

Motion sequence:

First the supporting leg straightens, followed by the hip, and then the upper body. Within this sequence, the player uses the momentum of the kettlebell and arrives in the final position (see photo 260b).

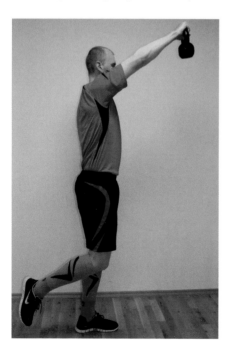

Final position:

Extend the body (legs, hip, upper body).

Next, move the kettlebell back into starting position with a quick but controlled motion and repeat the motion sequence. This exercise can also be performed with just one or both arms with secure footing.

Photo 260b

EXERCISE 2: UPRIGHT KETTLEBELL LATERAL RAISE

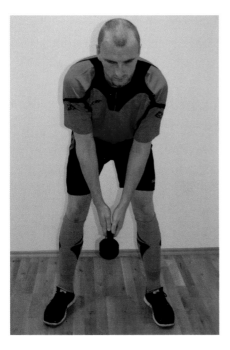

Starting position:

In a bent-over position (up to 90 degrees at the hips, depending on strength level), hold the kettlebell with both hands in front of the body.

Motion sequence:
Energetically raise the kettlebell to one side. Avoid static phases.

Photo 261a

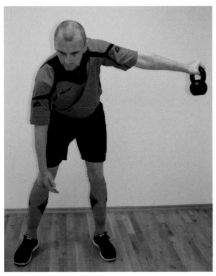

Final position (intermediate position):
You have reached the point of return when the arm is at chest level.

Next lower the kettlebell and use the generated momentum to switch hands at the lowest point, and raise the kettlebell on the other side. This motion sequence can also be performed in an upright position.

Photo 261b

EXERCISE 3: KETTLEBELL CIRCLES

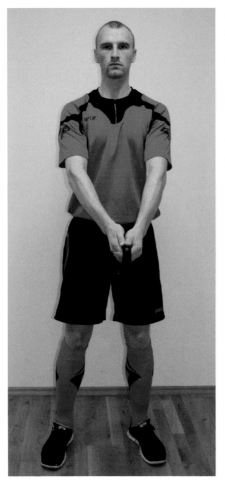

Starting position:
Stand upright and hold the kettlebell in front of the bodywith both hands.

Motion sequence:
Let the kettlebell circle the body with the arms extended. Always switch hands in the front and behind the back.

Photo 262

EXERCISE 4: KETTLEBELL FIGURE-EIGHTS

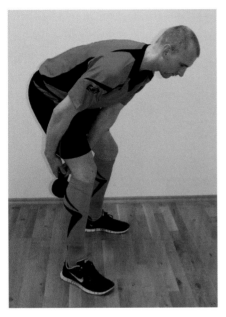

Starting position:
With knees slightly bent, hold the kettlebell between the legs with both hands. Head and back form a straight line.

Photo 263a

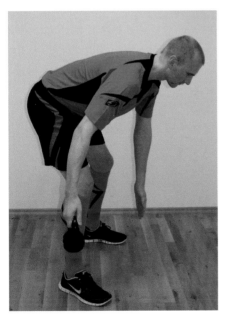

Motion sequence:
Move the kettlebell through the legs in figure-eights. Keep the back straight.

Photo 263b

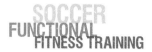

16.2.7 INDIVIDUAL ATHLETIC TRAINING THROUGHSLING TRAINING

Sling training includes anything that involves the use of ropes that are suspended from the ceiling or trees or attached to walls or posts. The advantage of this additional training method is that the ends of the ropes can move freely within two axes. By activating his muscles, the player can ensure a stable support surface.

Since deficiencies in core strength have been identified, particularly in youth competitive soccer, safeguarding resilience and the capacity for athletic exertionthrough appropriate versatile core training plays a leading role here.

Lowering injury risk and avoiding symptoms of overuse.

In a current empirical study, Riegler and Stöggl (2014, p. 20-23) were able to ascertain over a period of six weeks that core strength training with the sling trainer (in a stabile position) led to significant improvements in the muscle chains. They attributed these definite increases (compared to training on a stable support surface) to the greater sensorimotor neuromuscular adaptation through variable instability stimuli due to the higher demands being placed on the neuromuscular system. Sling training induces increased transmission of afferent information to the central nervous system, which in turn transfers more efferent neurons for motor control (see Taube, 2012).

Optimally developed maximum strength and power can only be converted to soccer-specific movements with core muscles that work effectively (Verstegen and Williams, 2006; Müller-Wohlfahrt and Schmidtlein, 2007; and Lüchtenberg and Görgner, 2010).

Sling training offers the greatest activation of proprioceptive systems (Magnuson et al., 1996), and in terms of additional perturbation[32], next to the balance board, vibration plates, air stability wobble cushion, and slacklining (see Meier, 2011),is meant to subsequently contribute to the optimization of ventral, lateral, and dorsal core muscle chains (local stabilizers) in performance training.

---

32   *The dictionary defines perturbation as interference/disturbance.*

Supplemented by sport-specific core training, sensorimotor neuromuscular training should be done regularly for at least 25 minutes a week to prevent joint injuries (especially in lower extremities) and to improve muscle strength, explosive strength, reaction time, and balance (Riegler and Stöggl, 2014, p. 23, and Behmand Anderson, 2006). The number of repetitions or the duration and number of series should be chosen according to training emphasis and the player.

Sling trainers are available commercially in different styles and at affordable prices. The authors' following exercises were performed in a professional fitness studio with the Dr. Wolff Functional Training[33] Station. These exercises can also be used to test core strength.

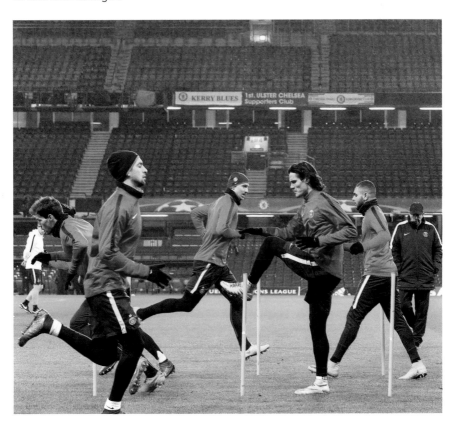

---

33 *In technical literature the term functional training has different definitions and interpretations. Bruscia (2015) recently presented a handbook on the subject in which he formulates the underlying training principle as follows: "The training of each motor property or skill must be programmed based on the action and function*

EXERCISE 1

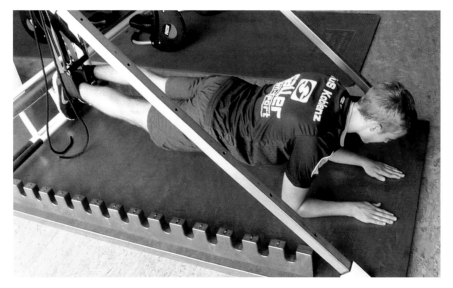

Photo 264: Get into a forearm plank position with the right leg in a sling.

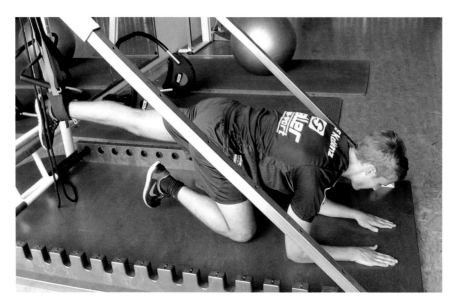

Photo 265: The free leg moves sideways toward the elbow and then back to starting position.
Keep the pelvis level. Avoid "whipping motions" of the lumbar spine!

EXERCISE 2

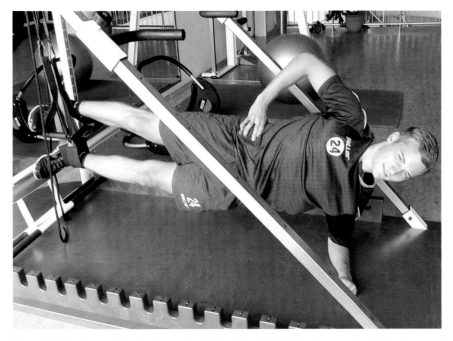

Photo 266: Perform a side plank to activate the lateral chain. One leg remains in the sling, and shoulders, pelvis, and knees are lined up. Lower and lift the pelvis from this position.

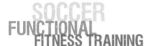
EXERCISE 3

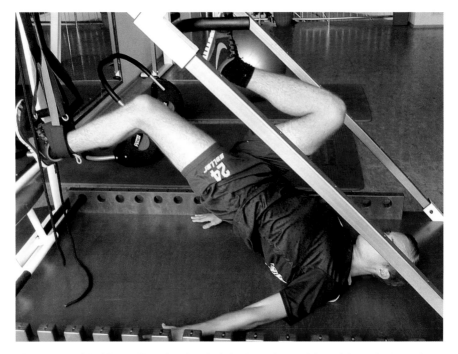

Photo 267: Pelvic lift: Working the dorsal chain in supine position with emphasis on lower extremities. One leg is pushed into the sling causing the hip to extend. Lift and lower the pelvis in one-second intervals.

EXERCISE 4

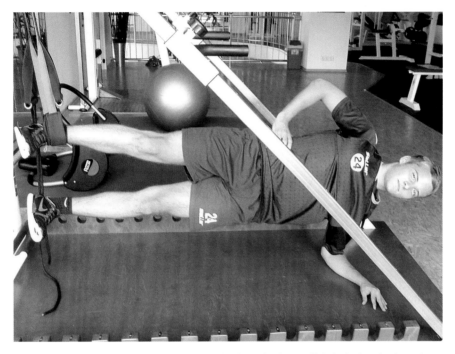

Photo 268: See exercise 2 for form.This side plank works the medial chain (emphasis on lower extremities). The upper leg presses into the sling with the inside edge of the foot, and the pelvis again lifts in one-second intervals.

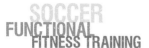

EXERCISE 5

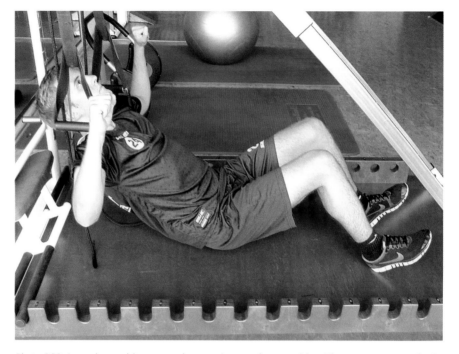

Photo 269: In supine position, move the arms into goalpost position. The upper arms rest in the slings. Here the emphasis is on the interscapular muscles.

EXERCISE 6

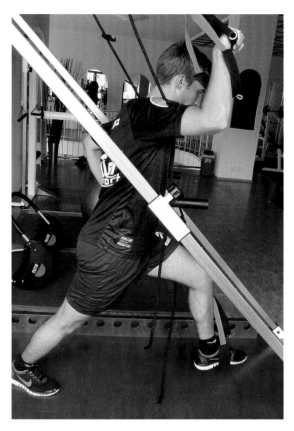

Photo 270: Lunge: The forward foot is placed in the sling with legs in a lunge position, and the back knee is lowered toward the floor with proper leg alignment. This exercise activates primarily the gluteal muscles, thigh muscles, and balance.

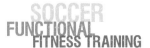

EXERCISE 7

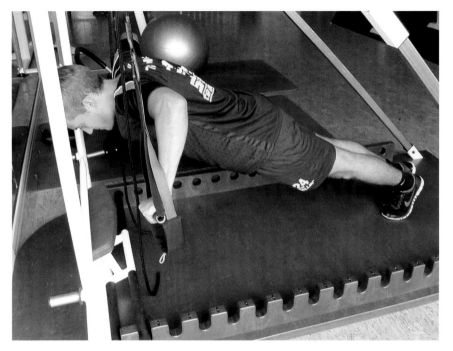

Photo 271: Push-up: Perform push-ups with hands in slings. This exercise works the ventral chains with emphasis on upper extremities.

16.2.8 INDIVIDUAL ATHLETIC TRAINING THROUGH CORE EXERCISES AND MOBILITY TRAINING

Core exercise, and this generally combines **core stability** and **core strength**, as part of rehabilitation has been empirically researched since the 1990s by Bermark (1989), Hodges et al. (1996), and Richardson et al. (1999). This initially resulted in rehab programs for patients with back problems. Since then the question of whether there is a significant link between good trunk stability and increased athletic performance has been—and still is—the subject of much research, which was summarized particularly by Gustedt (2013, p. 11-15).

In European soccer,**core performance** became known with Mark Verstegen in

2006, during the World Cup in Germany.[34] At this time, there are many published works on **core performance** in soccer training (Verstegen and Williams, 2006).

Therefore, the authors hereafter will focus primarily on a differentiated description of the terminology and target areas, the currently verified findings on core exercise and their bearing on soccer training, and their practical application.

The term **core** generally refers to the area between shoulders and knees (see fig. 62).

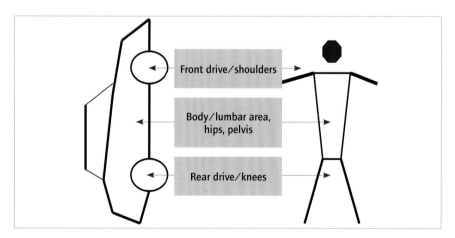

Fig. 62: High speed and stability go handinhand!

---

34   *Fitness coach of the German national soccer team under Jürgen Klinsmann.*

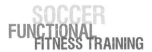

As shown in fig. 62 (compared to a car), the core muscles generate strength (as the basis for each movement), transfer strength from the upper to the lower extremities, and stabilize the spine. In the technical literature, the 29 participating muscles of the body's midsection are differentiated as **local** and **global muscle groups** and are summarized in table 14, based on Faries and Greenwood (2007, p. 12).

Table 14: Local and global muscle groups (modified based on Faries and Greenwood, 2007, p. 12)

Local muscles (Stabilizing muscle system)		Global muscles (Mobilizing muscle system)
Primary	**Secondary**	
Transverse abdominal muscle	Internal obliques	Rectus abdominus muscle
Back muscles	External obliques (medial fibers)	External obliques (lateral fibers)
	Quadratus lumborum muscle	Psoas major muscle
	Diaphragm	Erector spinae muscle
	Pelvic floor muscles	Iliocostalisthoracis muscle
	Iliocostalis of the lumbar region and erector spinae	

Of practical importance for **core exercise** on the training ground is that local (small and deeper muscles) muscles consist of **slow-twitch fibers** with 30-40% of maximum voluntary contraction, and global (large and exterior) muscles consist of **fast-twitch fibers** with more than 40% of maximum voluntary contractions. Both muscle groups work together synergistically and primarily help to stabilize the spine and allow the player to use a large range of motion.

Moreover, there is generally a functional difference between **core stability** and **core strength**. In training,**core stability** comes into play when a player must be in an optimal position during a physical movement. Here the aim is to control the movement of the trunk relative to the pelvis.

Core strength focuses on muscular control all around the lumbar spine. It enables the preservation of functional stability (Kibler et al., 2006; Faries et al., 2007).

Many different types of core training are used during practical training. Hereafter the authors will focus on exercises that target overall trunk stability and thereby ensure a high degree of physical resilience in soccer training to build up effective long-term performance. Furthermore, training volume and intensity go up considerably with increasing age in performance-oriented youth training so that injury prevention due to core training cannot be ranked highly enough by coaches and instructors. But here, too, it must be stated that pure core stabilization training does not lead to improved athletic performance in competitive soccer (Gustedt, 2014, p. 15).

With respect to practical training it should be emphasized here that static exercises are geared toward increasing strength and fatigue resistance of core muscles (primary stabilizers), and dynamic exercises (with small range of motion in back and pelvis) are geared primarily toward the development of secondary muscles.

As the following photo series will effectively show, here, too, individual athletic training through core exercise should be viewed as a kind of interface between strength abilities and target movements at the highest technical level (see chapter 1).

During a game, we soccer players are constantly faced with tasks that we want to complete successfully. **Core exercise** can help prepare us to do so!

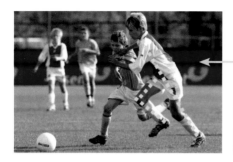

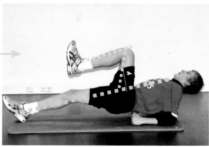

Photo 272: Core stability is a must!

Photo 273: We work hard for core stability.

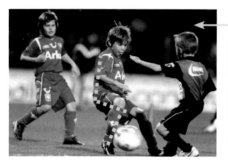

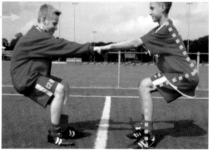

Photo 274: Complete balance!

Photo 275: Maintaining balance with a functional exercise.

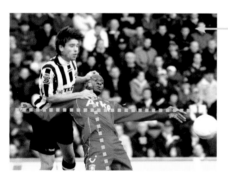

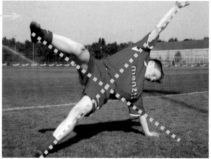

Photo 276: Staying balanced in all directions!

Photo 277: Maintaining muscle tension diagonally, too!

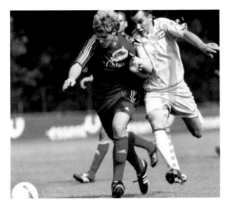

Photo 278: Lateral stability

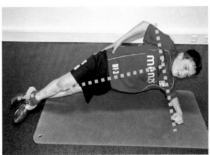

Photo 279: Lateral stability

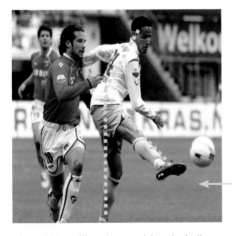

Photo 280: Agility when receiving the ball.

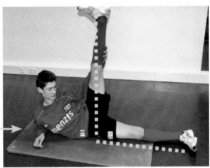

Photo 281: Hip mobility

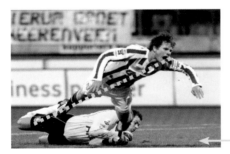

Photo 282: Falling without getting hurt.

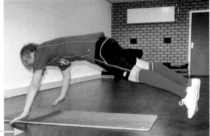

Photo 283: Pushing off and landing on hands and feet.

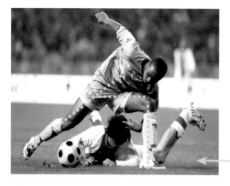

Photo 284: A deep side lunge requires lots of muscle elasticity.

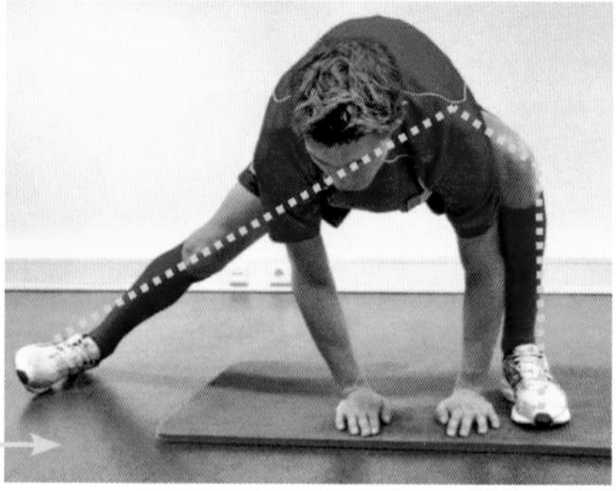

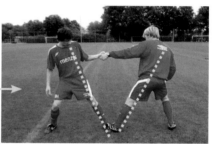

Photo 285: Adductor flexibility.

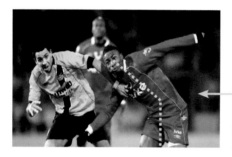

Photo 286: Regaining balance after being off-balance.

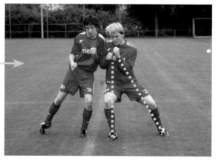

Photo 287: Dynamic stability helps maintain balance.

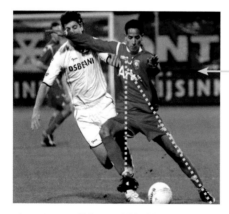

Photo 288: Colliding and blocking!

Photo 289: Shoulder to shoulder and maintaining balance.

In the following sections, the authors present different core packages for training U13/U12 to U19/U18 players.

16.2.8.1 TOP 12CORE EXERCISE PACKAGES FOR TRAINING U13/U12 TO U19/
U18 PLAYERS

In the following sections, the authors establish the direct link to practical training by introducing 12 **core exercises** for each of the U13/U12 to U19/U18 groups of players that can be performed without lots of equipment before, during, and after soccer practice. They can be supplemented with or substituted by the many exercises presented in this book. **Core exercise** should be a regular part of soccer fitness training. It provides important controlling elements with respect to compensation of muscular deficiencies, load regulation and stabilization, and mobilization. With different performance levels, goals, and training volumes and intensities, the number of training units per week can only be quantified with a general orientation mark (see also chapter 6;Fröhlich, Schmidtbleicher, and Emrich, 2007, p. 6-21).

Table 15: Benchmarks for training with core exercises in the context of training that includes preparatory and competitive periods in competitive soccer

Number of training units per week	Number of core exercises during preparatory periods	Number of core exercises during competitive periods (of the entire season)
2x for youth players and men/women	1 x	1 x
3 x for youth players and men/women	2 x	1 x
4 x for youth players and men/women	2-3 x	2 x
5 x and more for U13/U12	3 x	2 x
5 x and more for U15/U14	3 x	2 x
5 x and more for U17/U16	3 x	2 x
5 x and more for U19/U18	3-4 x	2-3 x
5 x or more for men/women	3-4 x	2-3 x

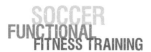

Table 16: Benchmarks for training content and methods for training with core exercises in competitive soccer

Teams/age groups	Stabilization and mobilization exercises for abdominal muscles	Stabilization and mobilization exercises for trunk musculature	Stabilization and mobilization exercises for shoulder and arm musculature
	Number of technically demanding executions per exercise		Rapid executions per exercise
U13/U12	10-12 x	10 x	6-8 x
U15/U14	12-14 x	12 x	9-10 x
U17/U16	14-16 x	14 x	10-12 x
U19/U18 and men/women	16-20 x	16 x	10-12 x

The **core exercises** in the following program affect the players very differently depending on training goal, individual, years of training, technical skill level, execution speed, training intensity and volume, and methodological choices. The authors, therefore, advocate for a high degree of individualization in the planning and implementation of **core exercises.**

16.2.8.1.1 CORE EXERCISES FOR U13/U12 PLAYERS

The authors suggest the following 12 core exercises for U13/U12 individual athletic training:

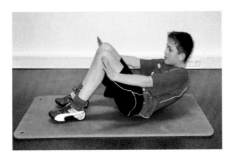

Photo 290: Sit-ups, and lift the upper body slightly by pushing forward with the palms.

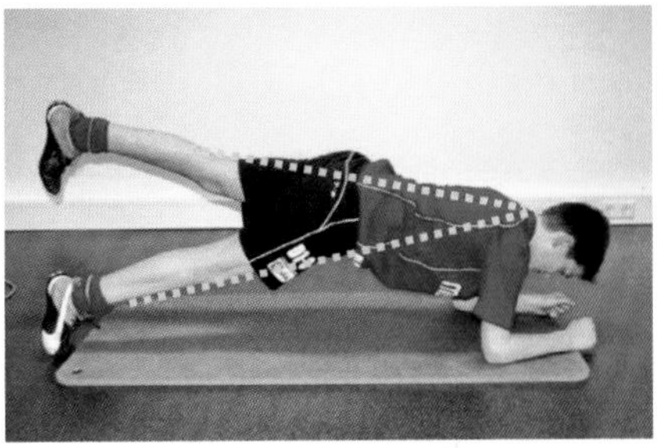

Photo 291: Forearm plank with one raised leg.

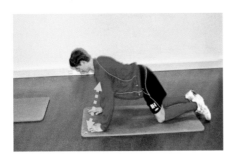

Photo 292: On all fours, pitch forward into plank and then vigorously push off.

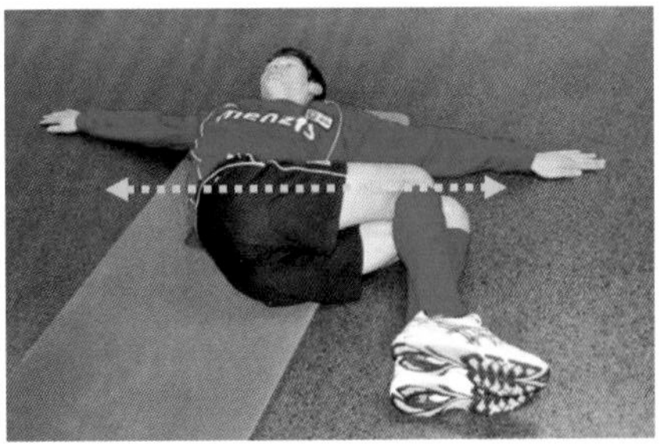

Photo 293: Windshield wipers with knees bent.

Photo 294: Cat–cow: Hold each pose for two seconds.

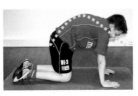

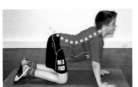

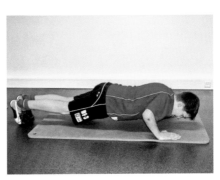

Photo 295: Plank at shoulder level.

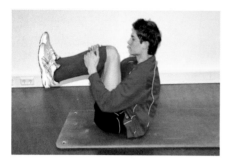

Photo 296: Jack-knife with knees bent.

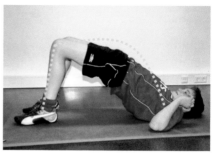

Photo 297: Move into bridge and hold it for two seconds.

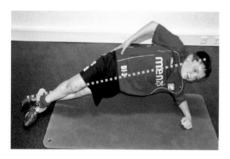

Photo 298: Side forearm plank with legs crossed.

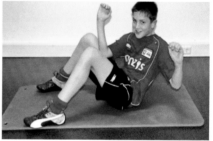

Photo 299: Diagonal sit-ups (only if abdominal muscles are already well developed).

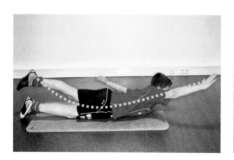

Photo 300: In prone position, raise one arm and one leg on a diagonal, alternating sides.

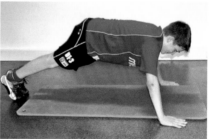

Photo 301: Wide push-ups (only if arm, shoulder, and trunk muscles are already well developed).

16.2.8.1.2 CORE EXERCISES FOR U15/U14 PLAYERS

The following 12 core exercises proved beneficial in U15/U14 practical training:

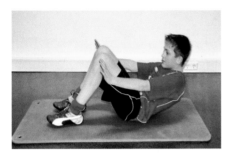

Photo 302: Sit-ups and lift the upper body slightly by pushing forward with the palms. Variation: Cross the arms in front of the chest.

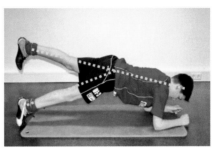

Photo 303: In a forearm plank, alternate raising one leg.

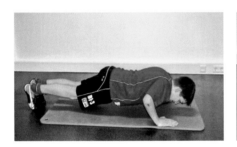

Photo 304: Push-up at shoulder level.

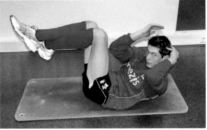

Photo 305: Diagonal crunches with legs crossed and raised.

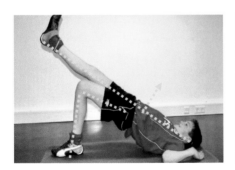

Photo 306: Pelvic lift: In supine position with one knee bent and the other leg extended upward, raise the posterior.

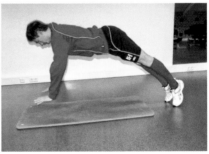

Photo 307: Concentric push-off and eccentric absorption of impact with hands and legs.

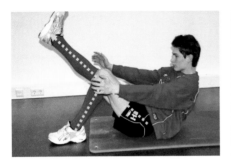

Photo 308: Perform sit-ups while alternately extending one leg.

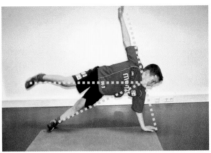

Photo 309: From a push-up position, switch to the position shown, extending arms and legs and balancing.

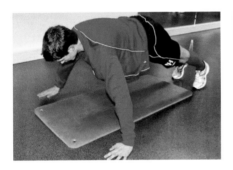

Photo 310: Wide push-ups: Bend and straighten the arms.

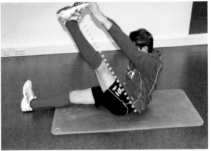

Photo 311: Single-leg jack-knife, alternating legs from a seated position with legs extended. (Only advanced athletes should perform this exercisedue to significant spinal cord compression.)

Photo 312: Child's pose to cobra, alternating in a two-second rhythm.

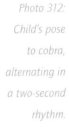

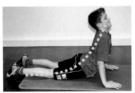

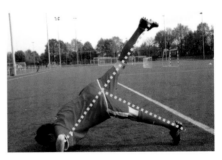

Photo 113: Perform push-ups with one leg extended at a near 90-degree angle in the final position.

16.2.8.1.3 CORE EXERCISES FOR U17/U16 PLAYERS

U17/U18 players are given 12 **core exercises** that are appropriate for their developmental level (measured in years of training).

See photo 302 of U15/U14 players: Sit-ups, lifting the upper body slightly by pushing forward with the palms.

VARIATION:

❂ Palms against the head.

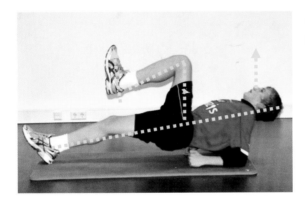

Photo 314: Marching in reverse forearm plank position.

See photo 301 of U13/U12 players: Wide push-ups.

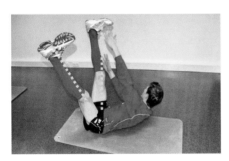

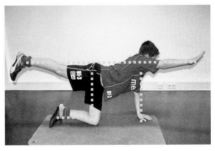

Photo 315a: Straddle jack-knife.(Only advanced athletes should perform this exercise due to significant spinal cord compression.)

Photo 315b: Diagonal movement on all fours: From a single-arm plank, extend one leg and one arm on a diagonal.

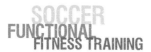
See photo 307 of U15/U14 players: Concentric push-off and eccentric absorption of impact with hands and legs.

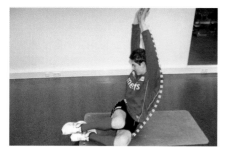

Photo 316a: From a supine position, bending at the hip joint and the knees, lift your extended upper body off the floor.

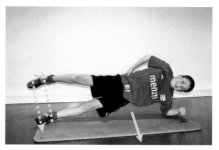

Photo 316b: Forearm side plank and raise the upper leg, and lift and lower the hips.

See photo 295 of U13/U12 players: Push-ups at shoulder level.

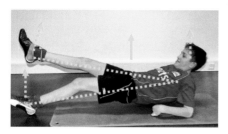

Photo 317a: Reverse forearm plank: Lift the hips and alternately lift and lower the legs.

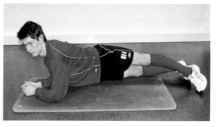

Photo 217b: Forearm plank: Cross your legs and try to touch the mat with your hip.

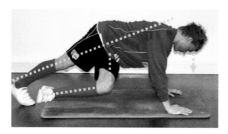

Photo 318: Perform push-ups at shoulder level with simultaneous internal rotation of one bent knee between mat and body.

16.2.8.1.4 CORE EXERCISES FOR U19/U18 PLAYERS

U19/18 players want coaches and instructors to give them 12 **core exercises** that are in line with their training progression, and those exercises are presented here.

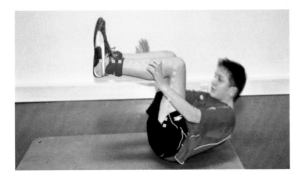

Photo 319: Balancing crunches with knees bent.

See photo 314 of U17/U16 players: Marching in reverse forearm plank position.

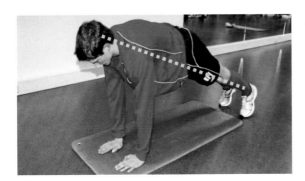

Photo 320: Narrow push-ups.

See photo 305 of U15/U14 players: Diagonal crunches with legs crossed and raised.

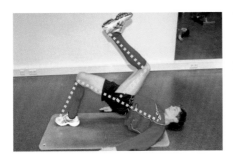

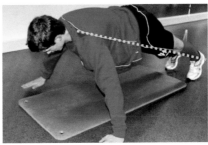

Photo 321a: Supine position with pelvis lifted and one leg extended up with knee bent.

Photo 321b: Wide push-ups.

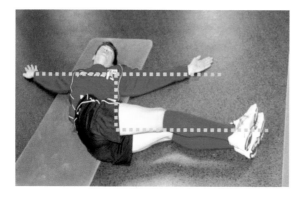

Photo 322: Windshield wipers: Legs do not touch the floor.

See photo 316 a of U17/U16 players: From a supine position, bending at the hip joint and the knees, lift your extended upper body off the floor.

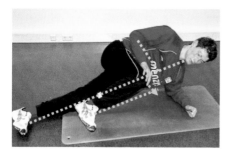

Photo 323a: Perform a forearm side plank, pulling the top knee in at a 90-degree angle.

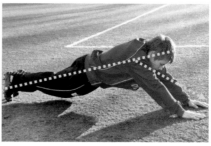

Photo 323b: Perform forward-shifting push-ups.

Photo 324: In a forearm side plank, continuously alternate moving the top leg in front and behind the supporting leg.

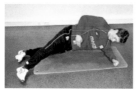

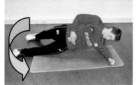

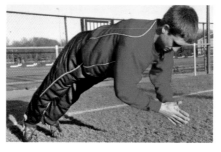

Photo 325: Push off from a push-up position, clap your hands, and land softly back in push-up position.

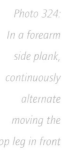

348

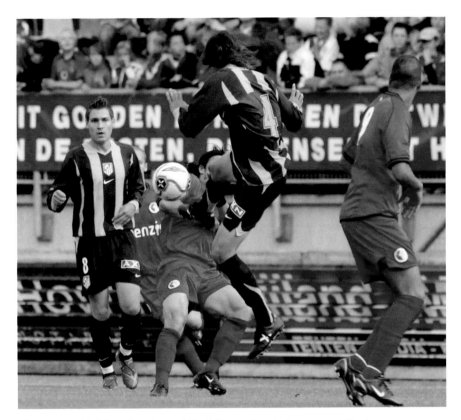

Photo 326: Athleticism, dexterity, and flexibility overlap during a competition!

The listed **core exercises** should be modified with the addition of supplementary equipment within the context of ambitious performance training and within the scope of a long-term training process. It is a way to break up routines that often result in disinclination to practice and performance stagnation. Explaining the many variations to the previous core exercises would go beyond the scope of this book.

We will briefly mention just a few: **core training** with the Deuser Band or Thera-Band and a medicine ball; fascial stretch training with a roller; stabilization training with the BOSU ball, the balance board, and different vibration plates; and rope training with ropes of different weights. Here we refer the interested reader to the following topical sources that have been tried and proven so far: Braun (2014); Geisler (2013 and 2014), and Schiffers (2014).

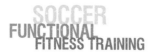
16.3 A DIFFERENT APPROACH TO FAIR TACKLING AND WHOLE-BODY TRAINING IN SOCCER[33]

(With assistance from Detlef Herborn and Eduard Feldbusch)

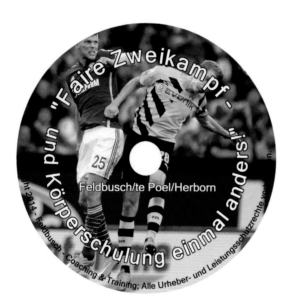

At first glance, soccer and Judo appear to have nothing in common to us soccer coaches and instructors. Moreover, many of our colleagues are told right away that leg acceleration must be taught only so the referee can point, for instance, to "the spot" in the penalty box. So how does Judo training for soccer players make any sense?

As was already thoroughly analyzed in chapter 7, two-thirds of all injuries in soccer occur during physical contact (Schmitt, 2013, p. 18-27).

Judo is one of the most physically and mentally demanding martial artsand is considered a combat sport in duel form that focuses particularly on versatile training in its training plan (see chapter 8). Judo will

- ❯ expand the movement experience and cognitive ability,
- ❯ intensively train fitness-related performance in competition (particularly coordination abilities like balance, orientation, and reaction), and
- ❯ developassertiveness during direct physical contact.

---

33 *For DVDs and information go to http://feldbusch-cat.de/fussball/judo-im-fussball.html and at Meyer & Meyer Sport. This topic was also treated by te Poel/Herborn (2015, p. 9-14) for practising school sports.*

Judo emerged in the late 19th century as a recreational sport for Japanese students dealing with lots of one-sided mental pressure. Jigoro Kano removed all the dangerous and strictly self-defense holds from jiu-jitsu and developed a one-on-one combat sport with specific rules. Today, judo can be found in the curricula of many governmental departments of education under the category "wrestling and grappling by rules—one-on-one combat sport".

From the perspective of youth competitive sports, the comprehensive strengthening of the musculoskeletal apparatus through judo is especially important during childhood and adolescence. In addition, judo training can also have a positive effect on dueling behavior (also and particularly in terms of an authoritative attitude toward oneself and the opponent).

Before a judoka is allowed to compete against another fighter he must demonstrate his judo skills in a test that includes falling techniques. In judo, two skills are basic requirements for an injury-free bout:

1. Throwing well (Nagekomi).
2. Falling well (Ukemi). Someone who is able to fall well is not tense and, therefore, less afraid in a bout. That is why lots of emphasis is placed on the principles of falling techniques. Learning protective motion sequences within the scope of a falling technique is meant to prevent frequent joint injuries to shoulders, elbows, hands, or knees. This provides a direct link to the chosen athletic training in soccer.

Furthermore, the surface of the judo mat (tatami) makes it possible to incorporate gymnastic elements and acrobatic exercises into training.

The authors would like to direct interested coaches and instructors to http://feldbusch-cat.de/fussball/judo-im-fussball.html for specific information (including a DVD and planned training courses on-site) on the use of judo exercises in youth and competitive soccer training.

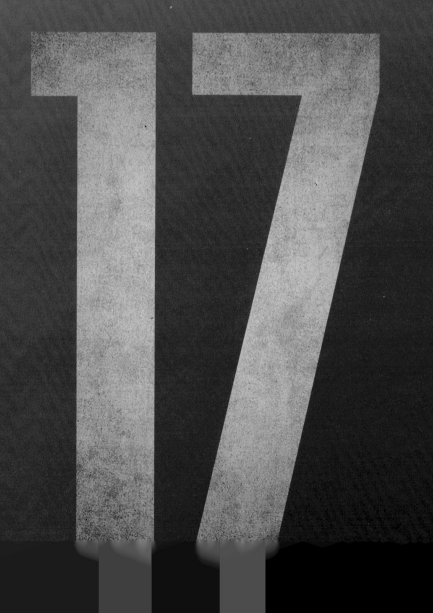

CHAPTER

17

17 COORDINATION AND SPEED TRAINING FOR SOCCER PLAYERS – FROM MULTITASKING STRATEGY TO BATTLE TRAINING

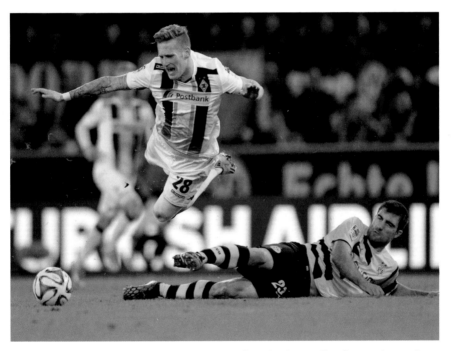

In modern youth soccer, the development of optimal coordination and speed are magic words for the future success of the forceful, relentlesslyoffensivemindset of emerging pro soccer players (Hartmann, 2004, p. 89). But how to build up these basic performance factors within a long-term development process and how to purposefully aim for them? We will now consider this question from a practice-oriented perspectivethat ties into chapters 3 and 4.

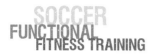

Based on their decades-long studies (including many projects in game sports, such as with TSG 1899 Hoffenheim), the Heidelberg, Germany, game sports researcher Dr. K. Roth and the Cologne, Germany, cognition and game sports researcher Dr. D. Memmert suggest working on a continuum between generality (e.g., jumping, skipping) and specificity (e.g., with a view to the movement task, foot-planting technique while dribbling) for the development of the performance factor, coordination, and to initiate, develop, and optimize this successive and/ or in concentric circles coordination during the training process (see fig. 63). The coordination-demanding training plan can be implemented *systematically* by

- changing the external conditions (environment, equipment),
- modifying the execution of movements (speed, amplitude, frequency),
- combining movement skills (vertical jumps with additional tasks such as squat or straddle),
- practicing under all pressure conditions (see table 18),
- modifying information assimilation (light conditions, noise),
- practicing at high intensity (heart rate, duration), and
- practicing under mental pressure (spectators, friends, opponents). (See Hohmann, Lames, and Letzelter, 2002, p. 112-113).

Table 17: Coordinationpressure in soccer [35]

Pressure of time
Pressure of precision
Pressure of sequential movements
Simultaneous pressure
Pressure of variability
Stress and strain

---

35   For more details see Weineck, Memmert, and Uhing, 2012, p. 67.

17.1 SYSTEMATIC COORDINATION TRAINING FOR SOCCER PLAYERS

When working on performance planning foryouth soccer, the following systematics can be used for the development of the performance factor coordination:

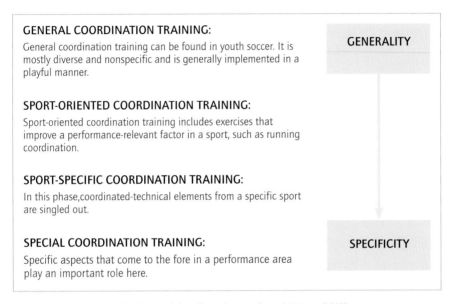

GENERAL COORDINATION TRAINING:
General coordination training can be found in youth soccer. It is mostly diverse and nonspecific and is generally implemented in a playful manner.

GENERALITY

SPORT-ORIENTED COORDINATION TRAINING:
Sport-oriented coordination training includes exercises that improve a performance-relevant factor in a sport, such as running coordination.

SPORT-SPECIFIC COORDINATION TRAINING:
In this phase,coordinated-technical elements from a specific sport are singled out.

SPECIAL COORDINATION TRAINING:
Specific aspects that come to the fore in a performance area play an important role here.

SPECIFICITY

Fig 63: Systematic coordination training (based on Roth and Kröger, 2011)

This will help thin out the general jungle of suggestions regarding coordination training and will allow the performance factor to be targeted resolutely during the training process through appropriate didactical and methodological decisions.

When starting general coordination training with the youngest players (ages seven to 13), cognitive abilities, information processing, attention span, and creative play,in particular, should be boosted in this age and developmental group, as it is done at the previously mentioned *Ballschule Heidelberg* (Ball School Heidelberg).

It can be considered empirically proven that well-developed coordination abilities have an extremely positive effect on learning new things, the quality of that learning, and its variable and situational availability (building-block ability-oriented ball school; Roth and Kröger, 2011). This boosting follows a *multitasking strategy*

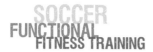

and is of fundamental importance since children have reached nearly 80% of their final performance level at the end of elementary school.[36]

When following the system in fig. 63, coordination training at this point is a kind of link to the power component speed (and technique). At first glance, from a perspective view, it is surprising that speed training could play a seemingly minor role in modern soccer given the (fast) *running distances without* the ball of .5 to 11% of the total running distance during a 90-minute game (Schlumberger, 2006, p. 125).

But a second look leads to the recognition that in today's elite soccer, under the aspects of *winning and defending the ball* as well as *scoring and preventing goals at a fast pace* (in addition to transitions,and here we must pay particular attention to the coordinated-technical links), the motor skill power component speed does nevertheless represent a performance-determining factor for successful action while competing (see chapter 4). Thus, at this point, running coordination (as sport-oriented coordination training) is being taken into account in youth soccer training.

As was previously explained in chapters 9 to12, the required qualifications for speed training (here in the form of running coordination) must absolutely be considered and acquired in advance:

- Basic forms of movement, such as jumping, crawling, rolling, hopping, pulling, pushing, grappling, throwing, falling, swerving, and stumbling
- Adequate strength potential
- Well-developed whole-body balance and stability
- Muscle elasticity

---

36 *Many practical training suggestions can be found in Roth and Kröger, 2011; Roth, et al., 2013; Roth, et al., 2014; Roth, Roth, and Hegar, 2014.*

17.2 SPORT-SPECIFIC COORDINATION TRAINING – THE ABCS OF RUNNING

Once one's "backpack" has been filled to the top with general coordination training, we move on to the running ABCs, which are characterized by skipping, high-knee running, leaping run, and ankle work and form the basis for economical and functional sprinting (see table 18):

Table 18: Running ABCs for soccer players (based on Grosser, 1991, p. 107-108) [37]

No.	Exercise	Execution/observation	Correction
1	Bouncy run on the balls of the feet	• Medium frequency • Active/reactive planting of the ball of the foot relative to the body's center of gravity (CG)	• If the toe is hanging down • If the calf whips forward • If leg and hip extension is insufficient
2	Bouncy leaps on the balls of the feet	• Slight knee lift • Active/reactive planting of the free leg relative to the CG	• If leg and hip extension is lacking • If the toe is hanging down
3	Bouncy run and bouncy leaps on the balls of the feet with single and double arm circles, forward and backwards	• Shoulders are relaxed. • Arm circles only out of the shoulder joint • No lateral pelvic twist	• If the shoulder is raised • If arms circling in running direction are not held close to the body
4	Bouncy run and leaps on the balls of the feet with alternating arm circles, forward and backwards	• Coordinated alignment of arms and legs (loose) • Active corresponding movement of arms and legs without lateral twisting	• If leg range of motion is not used during leg extension, and • When arms move at an angle to the running direction
5	Ankle work (AW) • Normal rate • Fastest rate • Increasing rate	• Minimal knee lift during active planting of the ball of the foot in direction of the CG • Active/reactive planting of the ball of the foot	• If the knee lift is too low or too high • If joints in legs do not extend sufficiently • If the toe hangs down and the ball of the foot is planted in front of CG
6	Ankle work with alternating upperleg raises (right and left)	• First extension, then active/reactive planting with weight shifted forward • Active support through coordinated arm movement	• If extension is insufficient • Ifthe ball of the foot is inactively planted with forwardsupport in front of the CG

---

37 *Additional examples, including grass running, for the interested reader can be found at*

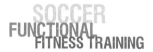
No.	Exercise	Execution/observation	Correction
7	Skipping (SK) • Normal rate • Fastest rate • Increasing rate	• Medium knee lift • Active/reactive planting of the ball of the foot in direction of CG • Leg and hip extension	• If extension is insufficient within range of motion • If the ball of the foot is actively planted with forward support • If the running posture changes during the transition to a run
8	*Alternate between ankle work and skipping* • Normal rate • Fastest rate	• *Immediate transition from AW to SK*	• *Review the individual phases if coordination of both elements is insufficient*
9	*High-knee run (HKR)* • High-knee lift • High-knee lift with forward movement of the calf Frequency can and must be modified in both versions.	• *Extension, forward lean, arm movement in running direction* • *Active/reactive planting with forward support in direction of the CG* • *Arm–leg coordination without lateral twisting of the upper body*	• *If knee lift is insufficient* • *If extension is lacking* • *If forward movement and planting of calf/ball of foot is passive*
10	*Skipping with transition to a run*	• *Coordinated transition of both exercise elements*	• *If coordination is lacking*
11	*Butt kick* • One side • Alternating sides • Alternating with transition to a run	• *Fast* • *Move thighs back slightly* • *Active/reactive planting with forward support* • *Coordinated arm and elbow movement in running direction*	• *If coordination is lacking* • *If the toe hangs down* • *If coordination is insufficient* • *If the ball of the foot is inactively planted with forward support*
12	*High-knee skips* • Horizontally with transition to a run	• *Extension of leg and hip joints* • *Coordinated arm support* • *Active/reactive planting* • *Upper extremities move in running direction*	• *If extension is lacking* • *If free leg activity is passive* • *If transition to a run is uncoordinated*
13	*Alternating jumps* • Vertical or horizontal with transition to a run	• *Knee extension and direction* • *Active/reactive planting of free leg in direction of the CG* • *Coordinated overall movement*	• *If extension is lacking* • *If activity into forward support is passive* • *If arm movement is uncoordinated*
14	*Running jumps* • With frequency • With transition to a run		

17.3 SPORT-SPECIFIC COORDINATION TRAINING FOR SOCCER PLAYERS

Moving along the continuum toward specificity in the training process (see fig. 63), another kinesiological perspective on coordination training can again provide an important grid analysis for soccer practice: sport-specific coordination training "[...] not stereotypical, mindless or abstracted repetitive motion, but [...] motivated and focused, diverse movement [...] can help coaches and instructors develop technical-coordinated elements in soccer (A/N)" (Neumaier and Mechling, 1999, p. 87).

Digression: For the planning of coordination training, Weineck, Memmert, and Uhing (2012, p. 99) suggest a tabular summary of the most important aspects of a planned movement task. Followingis a fragmentary outline (see table 19) of an example for running and jumping coordination, here the running ABCs (open stretch without ball; see table 20).

Table 19: Sample of a tabular summary for the planning of general running coordination without a ball, using the example of the running ABCs (based on Weineck, Memmert,and Uhing, 2012, p. 198)

Pressure conditions	Requirement profile	Coordination abilities	Movement task/technique	Degree of difficulty
Pressure of diversity	Gross motor skills (involves more than one-seventh of skeletal muscles) is kinesthetic.	Balance, orientation, adaptability, and rhythm	Running	Easy, moderate, difficult

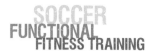

This makes training design, particularly in youth soccer, detailed, systematic, and highly practical.

For planning long-term soccer training, it is, therefore, extremely important to stress that soccer requires distinct (general and sport-oriented)coordination skills to make the fluid transitions between running and technical requirements flexible and harmonic (see chapters 3 and 4). These elements provide the basis for *sport-specific coordination training*, and soccer coaches and instructors often use them in exemplary combinations when desiring the use of both feet.

In the authors' opinion, this **training intentions** hould again become a greater focus in youth training in the future.

By now, *sport-specific* (and also *general and sport-oriented*) coordination training (with the ball) in basic youth soccer training (Roth and Kröger, 2011) is implemented around the world through

- *playsituation-oriented* (with team play, signaling availability and orienting, creating advantages, and evading opponent interference),
- *ability-oriented* (particularly with pressure of time, precision, diversity, complexity, and mental pressure), and
- *skill-oriented ball schools* (with getting open, keeping an eye on running lanes, playing angles, and controlling effort).

Not only are coordination abilities and skills trained, but alsoare the use of general tactical and technical modules.

The following modules represent content for beginning players in the area of coordination abilities:

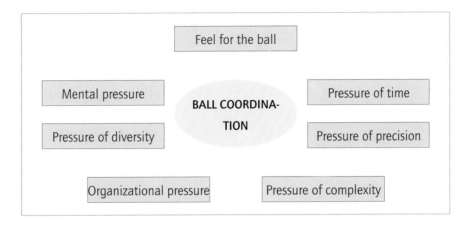

These can be combined with coordination tasks and follow the systematic formula:

Practicing coordinationmodules = simple technical tasks

+ difficult (general) coordinationtasks (pressure conditions)

Following is a practical example to elucidate the intrinsic system and focus of such coordination training in soccer (with the ball). [38]

---

38 *Interested readers can find many practical exercises and training examples for soccer training in te Poel and Hyballa (2015, p. 22-49).*

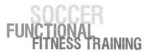
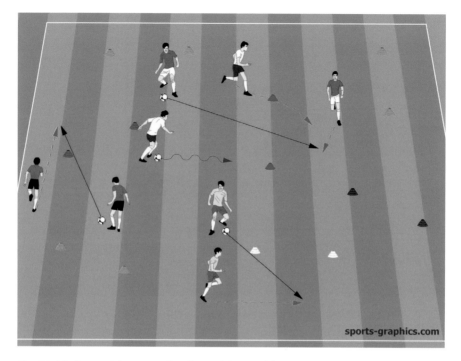

Fig. 64: Mission goal hunt—coordination training modules—passing through open goals with pressure of time and diversity

SETUP AND PROGRESSION:

- Form several player pairs, each with one ball.
- Set up goals with colored cones on any size field.
- The ball must be passed from a dribble through a cone goal into the partner's path.
- Points for goals scored must be counted out loud.
- Use stopwatch, extra balls, and possibly colored bibs.

VARIATIONS:

- Passing play with inside or outside foot or instep.
- Competitions: See which pair scores the most goals within a certain amount of time, or who needs how long to score10 goal points.
- Team competition: Two colors pass the ball back and forth through the goals. See which color pair (e.g., blue and yellow) are able to complete all possible combinations and possible goals in how much time.

In advanced and transition training and in competitive and elite training, coordination training often takes on the function of *supplementary coordination training* or *special coordination training*. Here it is used primarily to optimize certain important performance components (e.g., stride frequency) and currently to optimize cognitive and decision-making processes in soccer (Lutz, 2010) separately or in combinations, under the term life kinetics.

17.4 ACQUIRING A SOCCER-SPECIFIC RUNNING TECHNIQUE

The characteristic soccer running style, which is clearly different from track and field sprinting in terms of speed, represents one of these *special coordinated training* learning phases. In practice, it usually follows shortly after running coordination training and focuses on the following aspects of soccer:

- Soccer players rarely sprint in a straight line.
- Sprints in soccer are characterized by many and quick directional changes.
- Fast running in soccer always includes tempo changes.
- Most often a sprint in soccer involves an opponent and physical contact.
- Next to the appropriate physical effort, a sprint duel requires mental strength ("I want to win the ball and won't let the spectators' noisy reaction negatively affect me!").
- Sprint distances in soccer constantly vary between approximately 5.5 to 38 yards (5-30 m).

With respect to running technique, soccer players usually have a low center of gravity and minimal knee lift. "The low center of gravity and the associated forward trunk position appear to be advantageous to the soccer player with respect to constant readiness for a quick change in a current action (e.g.,taking the ball from the opponent, varying running speed, directional changes, tackles)" (Lutz, 2010, p. 126).

It has been the authors' experience in using a running technique that matches a biomechanical ideal that a player's individual running and movement style should not be broken. Rather, during a long-term training process,pay attention to gradually developing technical suggestions through running training units (see table 18) that

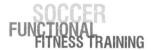
help develop a functional and economical running technique in soccer. In doing so, the following coaching aspects definitely come to the fore of self-correction and correction by someone else in practical training:

- Relax your head muscles.
- Relax your shoulders.
- Don't squeeze your breath, and don't tilt your head back.
- Lean slightly forward withyour upper body.
- While sprinting, swing your arms up to chin level.
- Keep your arms close to your body and at right angles.
- Move your feet vigorously toward the ground.
- Keep dynamic, "pointy" knees.
- Use reactive, active landing on the balls of the feet.

Translated to the speed in a soccer game, meaning the optimal relationship between passing length and passing frequency, the authors recommend the following rule of thumb for soccer training (which is always dependent on the respective game situation):

Speed = passing length x passing frequency

Within the scope of *special coordinatedor supplemental technical-coordinated training*, the special running and coordination exercises (without the ball) are characterized by five basic techniques:

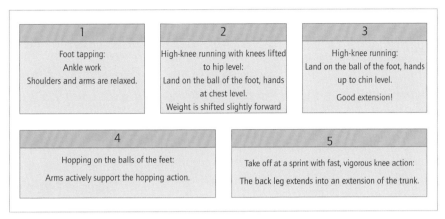

Fig. 65: Basic techniques for special running and coordination exercises (without the ball)

Based on the running ABCs(sport-oriented coordination training) and tables 18 and 19, these five basic techniques can be practiced in many different ways (also see exercises presented in Schöllhorn, 2003, p. 66; Lühnenschloss and Diercks, 2005, p. 105-148; Bauersfeld and Voss, 2007, p. 117-216). The authors recommend first eliminating *spatial movement errors* and then optimizing the *movement dynamic*. A *systematic approach* in the sense of a *differentiated learning approach* (Schöllhorn, 2003, p. 60-62) has been tried and tested. For practical training, this means

- focusing on individual aspects of the total movement,
- keeping practice conditions constant at first and then varying them, and
- bringing awareness about error sources through contrasting (i.e., exaggerated) movements and changing the outer boundary conditions (e.g., changing small obstacles).

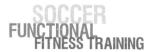

17.5 FOUR-WEEK COORDINATION AND SPEED TRAINING WITHOUT A BALL

So what could, for instance, a *four-week coordination and speed training* in youth soccer without a ball *within the warm-up phase* in soccer training regularly look like?

Fig. 66: The four-week coordination and speed stepladder

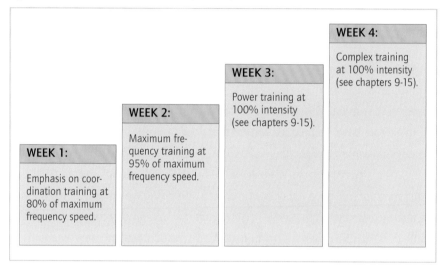

WEEK 1:
Emphasis on coordination training at 80% of maximum frequency speed.

WEEK 2:
Maximum frequency training at 95% of maximum frequency speed.

WEEK 3:
Power training at 100% intensity (see chapters 9-15).

WEEK 4:
Complex training at 100% intensity (see chapters 9-15).

Table 20: Scheduled coordination and speed training (without a ball) in youth training (E = exercises; A, B, C, and D = U19/18 to U13/U12 youth teams)

Coordination and speed training for A (U19/U18), B (U17/U16), C (U15/U14), and D (U13/U12) youth players. All exercises are the same.	Phase	Week 1	Week 2	Week 3	Week 4
		E 1-2-3-4	E 1-2-3	E 1-2-3	E 1-2
	1	All Es 2 x	All Es 2 x	All Es 2 x	All Es 2 x
	2	2	2	2	2
	3	3	3	3	3
	4	3	3	3	3
	etc				

WEEK 1:

EMPHASIS ON COORDINATION TRAINING AT 80% OF MAXIMUM FREQUENCY SPEED

Exercise 1

D: Two series of 5-m ankle work
C: Two series of 6-m ankle work
B: Two series of 7-m ankle work
A: Two series of 8-m ankle work

Exercise 2

D: Two series of 5-m medium- to high-knee skips
C: Two series of 6-m medium- to high-knee skips
B: Two series of 7-m medium- to high-knee skips
A: Two series of 8-m medium- to high-knee skips

Exercise 3

D: Two series of 5-m high-knee skips
C: Two series of 5-m high-knee skips
B: Two series of 5-m high-knee skips
A: Two series of 5-m high-knee skips

Exercise 4

D: Two series of 4-m high-knee skips with transition to 6-m sprint
C: Two series of 4-m high-knee skips with transition to 7-m sprint
B: Two series of 4-m high-knee skips with transition to 8-m sprint
A: Two series of 4-m high-knee skips with transition to 10-m sprint

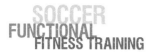

WEEK 2:

MAXIMUM FREQUENCY TRAINING AT 95% OF MAXIMUM FREQUENCY SPEED

Exercise 1

D: Two series of 3-m ankle work
C: Two series of 4-m ankle work
B: Two series of 5-m ankle work
A: Two series of 6-m ankle work

Exercise 2

D: Two series of 3-m medium- to high-knee skips and transition to 5-m sprint
C: Two series of 4-m medium- to high-knee skips and transition to 6-m sprint
B: Two series of 5-m medium- to high-knee skips and transition to 7-m sprint
A: Two series of 6-m medium- to high-knee skips and transition to 8-m sprint

Exercise 3

D: Two series of 3-m high-knee skips and transition to 5-m sprint
C: Two series of 4-m high-knee skips and transition to 6-m sprint
B: Two series of 5-m high-knee skips and transition to 7-m sprint
A: Two series of 6-m high-knee skips and transition to 8-m sprint

WEEK 3:

POWER TRAINING AT 95% INTENSITY (SEE CHAPTERS 13 AND 14)

Exercise 1

D: Two series of 3-m ankle work, 4 hops, and 5-m sprint takeoff
C: Two series of 3-m ankle work, 4 hops, and 6-m sprint takeoff
B: Two series of 4-m ankle work, 6 hops, and 7-m sprint takeoff
A: Two series of 4-m ankle work, 6 hops, and 8-m sprint takeoff

Exercise 2

D: Two series of 3-m medium- to high-knee skips, 4 hops, and transition to 5-m sprint
C: Two series of 3-m medium- to high-knee skips, 4 hops, and transition to 6-m sprint
B: Two series of 4-m medium- to high-knee skips, 6 hops, and transition to 7-m sprint
A: Two series of 4-m medium- to high-knee skips, 6 hops, and transition to 8-m sprint

Exercise 3

D: Two series of 3-m high-knee skips, 4 hops, and transition to 5-m sprint
C: Two series of 3-m high-knee skips, 4 hops, and transition to 6-m sprint
B: Two series of 4-m high-knee skips, 6 hops, and transition to 7-m sprint
A: Two series of 4-m high-knee skips, 6 hops, and transition to 8-m sprint

WEEK 4:

COMPLEX TRAINING AT 100% INTENSITY (SEE CHAPTERS 9-15)

Exercise 1

D: Two series of 2-m ankle work, 2-m medium- to high-knee skips, 2-m high-knee skips, 4 hops, and 5-m sprint
C: Two series of 2-m ankle work, 2-m medium- to high-knee skips, 2-m high-knee skips, 4 hops, and 5-m sprint
B: Two series of 2-m ankle work, 2-m medium- to high-knee skips, 2-m high-knee skips, 4 hops, and 5-m sprint
A: Two series of 2-m ankle work, 2-m medium- to high-knee skips, 2-m high-knee skips, 4 hops, and 5-m sprint

Exercise 2

D: Two series of 3-m hops and 5-m sprint takeoff
C: Two series of 3-m hops and 6-m sprint takeoff
B: Two series of 4-m hops and 7-m sprint takeoff
A: Two series of 4-m hops and 8-m sprint takeoff

The exercises should be varied constantly at practice and substituted with others from the running ABCs. The following can be variations of the previous exercises:

ANKLE WORK:

- Full rotation, left and right
- To the side and alternately left, right, and forward
- Backwards
- Backwards with full rotation, left and right
- Combine all of the ankle exercises with short sprints in all directions.

CHOOSE MEDIUM- TO HIGH-KNEE SKIPS:

- With full rotations, left and right
- In place
- Sideways
- Backwards
- Backwards with full rotation, left and right
- Sideways, left, right, and backwards
- Combine all of the medium- to high-knee skips with short sprints in all directions.

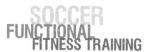

CHOOSE HIGH-KNEE SKIPS:

- With full rotations, left and right
- In place
- Sideways
- Backwards
- Combine all of the exercises with short sprints in all directions.

CHOOSE HOPS:

- 4 hops with full rotations, left and right
- Zigzag hops
- Hops in place
- Big hops to gain lots of space
- Big forward hop, small hop backward, and repeat
- High hop
- Short, quick hops, alternating with increasing height
- Backward hop with full rotation, left and right
- Combine all of the hop versions with short sprints in all directions.

BREAKING AWAY (AFTER A BALL-HANDLING TECHNIQUE):

- After a split stop
- After dribbling in place
- After a forward dribble
- After a backwards dribble
- After a jump
- After briefly hopping
- After high-knee skips to the left and right
- After a pass (the passing foot is the sprinting foot!).

17.6 EXAMPLES OF SPECIALIZED COORDINATION TRAINING

In youth soccer, the use of varied running and jumping tasksthat end with technical actions in the sense of *special coordination training or supplementary technical-coordinated training* is very important (Weineck, Memmert, and Uhing, 2012, p. 99). The authors provide several exemplary tasks here.

1. AGILITY LADDER AND SOCCER TECHNIQUES

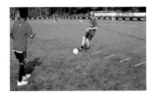 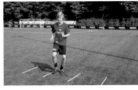 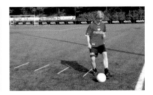

Photo 327a-c: Play the ball back with a flat pass. Move quickly sideways in a 1-2 rhythm and pass the second ball back (total: 10repetitions).

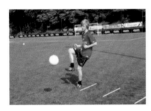 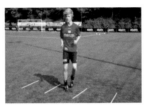 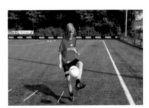

Photo 328a-c: Same as photo 327, but with a volley pass.

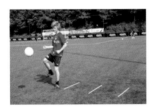 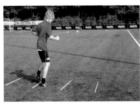 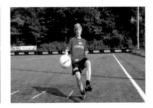

Photo 329a-c: Same as photo 327, but with quick rotation and a subsequent holding phase on one leg at the end of the ladder (stand and volley pass).

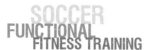

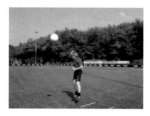
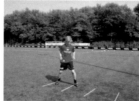
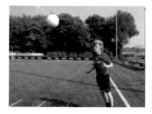

Photo 330a-c: Same as photo 327, but with header techniques from a jump.

2. KOMPLEXE FORMEN

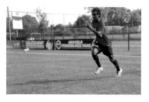
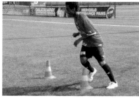
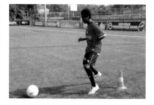

Photo 331a-c: Sprint 10 meters, decelerate, run a figure-eight between the cones, and play the passed ball back with a forceful flat pass.

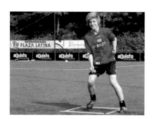
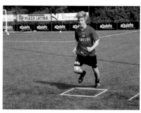
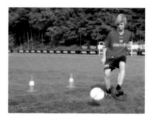

Photo 332a-c: Two players stand approximately 12 meters apart. The player in the square moves his legs very quickly forward and back, left and right, in a 1-2 rhythm. After a combination, the player in the square takes the initiative and breaks away. While running, he controls the ball passed by the second player and plays a precise return pass. The player who steps out of the square and sprints away chooses the moment the pass is played to him. Competition: See how far the player can sprint away before the pass reaches him. Setting up cones helps with quick orientation and determining the sprint distance.

Interested readers can find many additional running and jumping coordination exercises in Weineck and Uhing (2012, p. 197-216), and especially from the running and coordination coach, Hans Tanner (FC Zürich), the *Schnelligkeitszentrum* Berlin fitness center, and the Munich Youth Academy. For that reason, we only briefly reference the exercises in this book.

17.7 BATTLE FORMS – SUPPLEMENTAL TECHNICAL-COORDINATEDTRAINING WITH SPIRIT

A) KING OF THE FLAT PASS

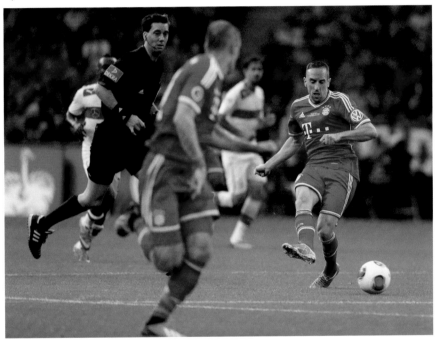

Photo 333: Ribery plays a flat pass.

Emphasis: Handling time pressure and precision and mastering the flat pass with both feet.

Task: Two players pass each other the ball with the wrong foot (left-footers use the right; right-footers use the left foot) at a distance of approximately 8 meters.

Competition rule: Both players start with 10 points. Each mistake (e.g., too hard or not precise) pointed out by the coach is penalized with a point deduction. Set time and point limits together.

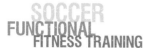
B) POSSESSION

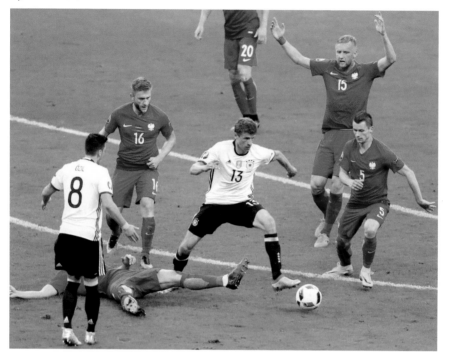

Photo 334: Thomas Mueller (C) of Germany ist surrounded by Polands Grzegorz Krychowiak (L-R), Jakub Blaszczykowski, Kamil Glik and Krzysztof Maczynski during the UEFA Euro 2016 match Germany and Poland

Emphasis: Handling time pressure while taking dribbling technique into account.

Task: One player dribbles in a marked space while being attacked by his partner, creating opponent pressure.

Competition rule: See who is able to dribble for 45 seconds without losing possession. Make charts and post them in the locker room. Choose duration and field size based on the training level.

C) SHOT ON GOAL

Emphasis: Time pressure and precision combined with the technique of a shot on goal.

Task: The player stands on the field surrounded by four mini goals and must shoot 10 passed balls into the mini goals with the wrong foot.

Competition rule: The coach counts the goals and establishes the quality criteria in advance (e.g., hard and flat). See who can score the most goals in 45 seconds. Make charts and post them in the locker room. Choose duration and field size based on the training level.

Additional variations for a) to c) include crosses with volley or header passes with goal player participation.

D) 1-ON-1

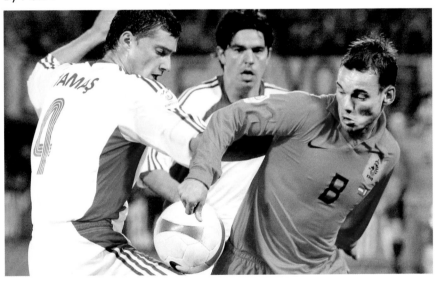

Photo 335: Dutch Midfielder Wesley Sneijder (r) in a duel against the Romanian Players Gabriel Tamas (l) and Cosmin Contra

Emphasis: Combine time pressure, precision, and complexity with shot on goal technique.

Tasks:

- Use the dribble approach and shot on goal at mini goals with opponent pressure (opposing player operates from the front and side or diagonally from the side).

375

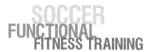

- ◉ The *shot on goal* is played with precision between the cones (cone posts) with and without opponent pressure.
- ◉ *Shot on goal* in direction of the goal with GP, in which the coach, who stands behind the goal, signals the direction of the shot.
- ◉ *Shot on goal* after a pass from a teammate. The player has his back to the goal and must score a goal.

Competition rule: The coach counts the goals and keeps a ranking list. Choose duration, repetitions, and field sizes based on the training level. Make charts and post them in the locker room.

E) FEINTS IN 1-ON-1

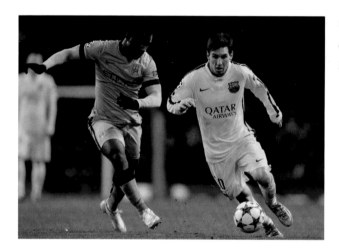

Photo 336: Lionel Messi dribbles around Wilfried Bony

Emphasis: Focus on subjective factors, variability, and time pressure, and use feinting techniques.

Tasks:
- ◉ Dribble across finish lines.
- ◉ Use Coerver Techniques: Zidane trick, Ronaldo trick, step-over, Beckenbauer turn, and Matthews move, for example.
- ◉ Evaluation by the coach or instructor is based on the famous figure skating scoring system: Ascore: goal or no goal; Bscore: quality of techniques (variability, esthetics, leg work).

Choose duration, repetitions, and field sizes based on the training level. Make charts and post them in the locker room.

The coach or instructor could design a **battle plan** as follows:

Table 21: Simple, individual battle plan for the season

For: Player X	Jersey number 5	Central defender (inside left)
Strong foot: left	6'1", 174 lbs.	Date of birth
Date	Emphasis: wrong foot (technique)	Winner (+)
Date	Emphasis: abdominals (athletics)	(−)
Date	Emphasis: wrong foot (technique)	Winner (+)
Date	Emphasis: defensive header (position)	(−)
Date	Emphasis: defensive header (position)	Winner (+)
Noteworthy: Slight induration in the left calf; therefore, no individual training possible!		
Date	Emphasis: trunk muscles (athletics)	(−)
Date	Emphasis: feints (technique)	(−)
Noteworthy: U19 training course (state selection), therefore, no individual training possible!		
Date	Emphasis: defensive header (position)	Winner (+)
Date	Emphasis: wrong foot (technique)	Winner (+)
Date	Emphasis: defensive header (position)	Winner (+)
Date	Emphasis: back muscles (athletics)	(−)
Date	Emphasis: precision shooting	Winner (+)
Date	Emphasis: back muscles (athletics)	(−)
Date	Emphasis: volleys (position)	(−)
Winter break until		
Date	Emphasis: defensive header (position)	Winner (+)
Date	Emphasis: wrong foot (technique)	(−)
Datum	Emphasis: wrong foot (technique)	(−)
Datum	Emphasis: wrong foot (technique)	(+)
Datum	Emphasis: feints (battle) (technique)	(−)
Datum	Emphasis: set pieces (technique)	(−)

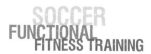

The recording of these elements as shown in the example is not very time-intensive and can be simplified by using a plus symbol (successful or winner of a team competition) and minus symbol. This provides the coach or instructor with a quick overview of the timeline and training level in this performance-limiting area, particularly at a youth high-performance training facility.

17.8 SPECIALIZED TRAINING CONTENT AND METHODS – WHAT ELSE WORKS?

In advanced and transition training and in competitive and high-performance training, speed training is often supplemented by additional forms of training.

Their purpose is to help improve specific elements of speed in soccer (without a ball):

- 20 and 50-meter sprints without load significantly improve **maximum speed** (Zafeiridis et al., 2005).

- Improve **time programs** with speed training using exercises with a jumping harness (Bauersfeld and Voss, 1992).

- Downhill sprints lead to a significant increase in **maximum speed** (Paradisis and Cooke, 1996).

- Maximum sprints (4 x 20 m and 4 x 50 m) with external resistance of 5 kilograms within the scope of an eight-week training program resulted in improved **sprint times** in 10-meter sprints (Zafeiridis et al., 2005).

- Combinations of vertical and horizontal jumps during training (including hurdles) lead to an improved **maximum speed** (Schlumberger, 2006, p. 127).

- Drop jumps lead to improved **stiffness** and **tension** in the lower extremities and, thereby, indirectly contribute to an increase in maximum speed. This factor is particularly relevant for youth players since they do not possess the required stiffness or tension in the pertinent musculature due to their developmental stage and level of training.

- Performance in the countermovement jump (CMJ) has a significant effect on sprint performance in 30-meter sprints.

- Speed bounding, a form of jumping with horizontal power output, appears to have a positive effect on improving **maximum sprint speed.**

- ❯ Ballistic training *(loaded jump squats)*contributes to a significant improvement in the **30-meter sprint.**

- ❯ Sprint acceleration (10-m distance) as well as maximum speed (20-m flying sprint) do not share any commonalities. This also applies to sprints with directional changes and linear sprints. Depending on the training goal, both must be trained separately (Wisloff et al., 2004).

- ❯ Vertical jump performance is representative of the power of the leg extensor muscle group. That is why "[...] traditional strength training with squats (hypertrophy method), power training with drop jumps and concentric squat jumps with added load (loaded jump squats) contribute to improved power" (Schlumberger, 2006, p. 128) and, thus,**maximum speed performance.**

- ❯ Norwegian pro soccer players were able to achieve significant gains in **vertical jump performance** (CMJ) through an eight-week strength training program with maximal power loads during squats (Schlumberger, 2006).

- ❯ "Weightlifting-oriented takeoff power techniques with high requirements for quick power output during complex coordination tasks (leg-trunk-arm coordination) can thus be classified as additional power-boosting methods" (Schlumberger, 2006). This statement applies especially to variations of the **clean and jerk.**

- ❯ A combination of strength and power training programs leads to maximum adaptations in power performance (Schlumberger, 2006).

- ❯ Active dynamic preparation strategies (**warming up** in the classic sense) have a more positive effect on subsequent speed and power performances (Schlumberger, 2006).

- ❯ Use **complex** or **contrast methods**. Here, deep squats with barbells, for instance, precede subsequent jumping and sprinting strength exercises. The effectiveness during submaximal and maximal exertion has been proven (Schlumberger, 2006).

- ❯ The effectiveness of jumping and sprinting strength training depends largely on the **maximization of intensities.** It can be actuatedin part through the players' motivation and willingness to exert themselves. Providing external goals (Can you catch the ball?) and immediate feedback regarding the performance (compared to the previous one: "Look at the display! You

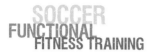

have never run this fast before!") can help to bring a positive aspect to the maximization of intensities during practical training.

● Integrating sprint and power training into the short- and long-term training structure:

a) A "[...] low-volume power training program (combining barbell exercises [squats, power cleans], vertical jumps, sprints)" leads "to an improved power performance" (Schlumberger, 2006, p. 130).

b) "It can therefore be concluded that relatively low-volume power and speed training programs for soccer players with a training frequency of 2-3 x per week within the scope of the overall training load can be considered adequate" (Schlumberger, 2006, p. 130).

When implementing these speed training elements, it is important to preserve the specifics of the target group. This means, forms of training for men and women must be kept separate from youth training. All in good time!

The key to sustainable training of performance-determining factors coordination and speed is still founded in a maximum amount of variability and in the many contact areas of the listed modules, and from there derives methodological approaches that, at times, are successive, differential, and concentric, and, thus, live down the stereotypical methods of the past.

CHAPTER

18

18 SOCCER FITNESS TODAY –HIIT BLOCKS, HIT PROGRAM, OR EMPHASIS ON INTERMITTENT LOADING?

> *"Soccer fitness is acquired by playing soccer. It is about using the right stimuli at the right time!"*

(Verheijen, 2009a, p. 26)

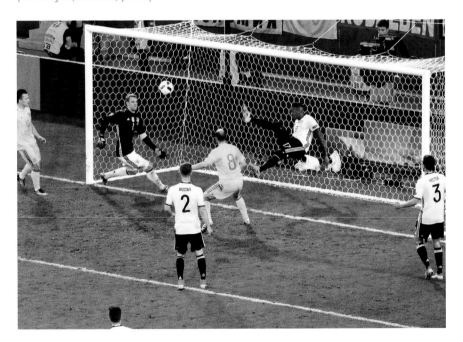

On that premiseand under the direction of head coach, Guus Hiddink, in 2008,

Dutch fitness trainer Dr. Raymond Verheijen began the three-week preparatory training of the Russian national soccer team for the European championships.

This periodization was preceded by fitness trainer Verheijen's practical experience with the different target-performance comparisons regarding "soccer fitness, regeneration, and explosive capacity" (Verheijen, 2009a, p. 29):

- Fitness trainer for the Dutch national team at the European championships in 2000 (with Frank Rijkaard; semi-finals) and in 2004 (with Dick Advocaat; semi-finals)
- Fitness trainer for the national teams of South Korea at theWorld Cup in 2002 (with Guus Hiddink; fourth place) and Australia in 2006 (with Guus Hiddink; round of 16)

Furthermore, Verheijen was able to implement the soccer fitness model with the club teams FC Barcelona, Feyenoord Rotterdam, and, since 2009, Manchester City. By using heart rate measurements from the *interval shuttle run test (ISRT)* and comparing them to previously ascertained results from senior European elite soccer and existing UEFA statistics, Verheijen was able to detect a definite drop in heart rate after major exertion with the end of exertion after 15- and 60-second rest periods in all players on the Russian national team at the start of the 2008 European championships. During the 2008 European championships, this resulted in "[...] our players being able to (N/A) run the most and sprint the most again in the semi-finals". (Verheijen, 2009a, p. 29). At the 2008 European championships, the Russian team made it to the semi-finals. The training exercises to improve soccer fitness consisted of 1-on-1 play (see fig. 67), 1-on-goal player (special training; see fig. 68), 1-on-0 plus cross against two attackers, 3-on-3 plus 2 goal players (see fig. 71), 4-on-4/5-on-5 plus 2 goal players (see fig 70), and 7-on-7/8-on-8 plus 2 goal players (see fig. 72) with ball and two goals with goal players. Verheijen added the power endurance training shown in fig. 69) (Verheijen, 2009a, p. 29).

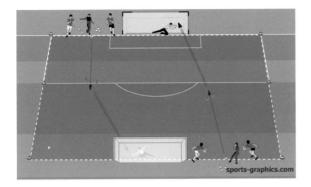

Fig. 67: 1-on-1—explosive power

PROGRESSION

- ❯ Double penalty area with two large goals and goal players.
- ❯ Player pairs stand to the right or left of each goal for 1-on-1-play. Between them is the coach or assistant coach with the ball.
- ❯ Controlled, straight *through pass* in the direction of the centerline.
- ❯ Both players take off after the ball to get a shot on goal.

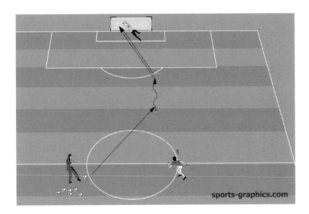

Fig. 68: 1-on-1 in the direction of the ball—sprint stamina (special training)

PROGRESSION

- ❯ The coach or assistant coach stands with the ball approximately 10-meters behind the centerline.
- ❯ The coach plays a pass in the direction of the goal with a goal player.
- ❯ The player chases the ball, controls the ball at top speed, and takes a shot as quickly as possible.
- ❯ Afterward, he jogs back.
- ❯ The coach directs the training load based on training level and training goal.

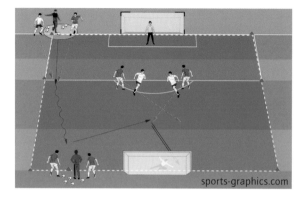

Fig. 69: Explosive power endurance—sprints with few passes

PROGRESSION

- Two crossing players face each other at the penalty area.
- Field size is 35 x 40 meters.
- 2 x 2 attacking players each are in the center (short-long; cross).
- The coach or assistant coach plays a straight *through pass* forward.
- Sprint to the ball and tempo dribble in the direction of the baseline with cross or return pass to two strikers.
- The coach directs the training load based on training level and training goal.

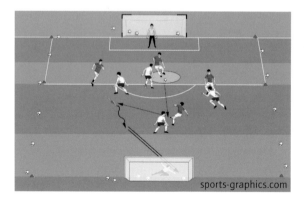

Fig. 70: 4-on-4 plus goal player/5-on-5 plus goal player

PROGRESSION

- 4-on-4 plus goal player/5-on-5 plus goal player on a field that is 40 x 35 meterswith two large goals.
- Both teams play in diamond formation to achieve a high overall running performance.
- Have lots of replacement balls ready next to sidelines and goals.
- The coach directs the training load based on training level and training goal.

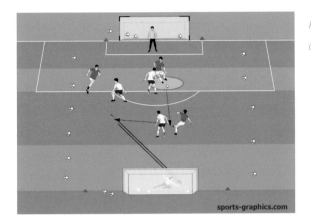

Fig. 71: 3-on-3—high speed and quick recovery

PROGRESSION

❯ 3-on-3 plus 2 goal players on two large goals on a field that is 30 x 20 meters.

❯ Keep up the pace.

❯ Have replacement balls ready.

❯ The coach directs the training load based on training level and training goal.

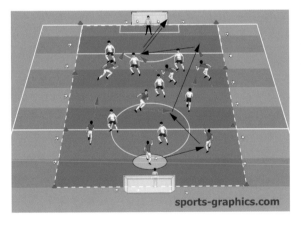

Fig. 72: 7-on-7 plus goal player/8-on-8 plus goal player—recovery endurance

PROGRESSION

❯ 7-on-7 plus goal player/8-on-8 plus goal player on two large goals on a field that is approximately 80 x 40 meters.

❯ Play several rounds with short breaks.

❯ Keep a fast pace.

❯ Keep replacement balls ready.

❯ The coach directs the training load based on training level and training goal.

Verheijen's 5-on-5 form of play (2009a) (goal player plus 4 against the goal player plus 4) is played on a field that is 40 x 35 meterswith two large goals (see fig. 70) and is a type of special form of play. Both teams play in diamond formation. Wide and deep coverage of the field and having lots of replacement balls at the ready ensures a significant running effort by the players. To make sure all players complete the same number of running repetitions, this type of "tempo periodization in forms of play" (Verheijen, 2009a, p. 30) can also be organized in the form of a tournament on two fields (e.g., 4 minutes exertion at high intensity and 3- to 5-minute rest). According to Verheijen, this form of play allows the coaches to

- keep a very close eye on the action,
- control the volume and intensity of physical exertion (e.g.,using heart rate monitors),
- make situation-appropriate changes with respect to technical–tactical emphases (superior or inferior number games and 8-on-8 on an appropriately larger field; see fig. 72),
- initiate the natural movement behavior of children and adolescents that is characterized by frequent, intermittently, highly intensive, and explosive movements (oscillating movement patterns), and
- take into consideration motivation and the joy of playing in competitive play.

Here the authors would like to stress that based on the opinion of Dr. Raymond Verheijen (2009b, p. 12),a lot of talent drops away, particularly in youth soccer, because "[y]oung players [...] are not (A/N) exposed to the physical demands step-by-step! That means fewer and shorter practices in the beginning, and fewer minutes of play. When pro players complete six training units per week, young talents don't need more than, for instance, four!" (2009b, p. 12). To Verheijen (2009b, p. 12), soccer fitness with the ball is part of a long-term plan that puts a slow buildup under special consideration of technical–tactical training units ahead of instant success.

To the authors, this aspect again points to the fact that Verheijen strives for a consistent philosophy for soccer training and instruction that is always closely based on competitive play and consistently derives its training content and methods from there. Thus, the philosophy of soccer fitness with explosive capacities and the periodization model (for men and women) persists, whereby training duration, volume, and intensity in youth training must be thought of very differently.

Soccer is a competitive sport with intermittent exertion. It is closely linked to speed, strength, coordination, and endurance, meaning the ability to repeat brief, highly intensive efforts during the game (Gahlul and Hofmann, 2015, p. 31-35).

By using this example from elite soccer, with the exclusion of the periodization and super compensation model, the authors want to show the youth player that according to Dr. Raymond Verheijen's (2009a and 2009b) body of knowledge and experience, the ball can be used consistently in soccer fitness training with properly coordinated forms of play—from basic, intermediate, and transition training up to advanced and high-performance training. In doing so,

- sport-related motor skill goals from the Dutch training philosophy,
- the development of technica–tactical abilities and skills all the way to sufficiently flexible use in interaction with teammates and opponents, and
- the development of action speed

can be transferred to advanced and high-performance training without any breaks in content and methodology.

Today, direct and indirect performance and development diagnostics and performance projections for endurance capacity[39] are done worldwide through different methods:

a) Directly: recording running performance
b) Indirectly: battery of fitness tests

---

39   *All endurance exercise under **normoxia** (normal oxygen supply) that leads to a decreased intracellular ATP concentration triggers an increase in aerobic capacity and increase in mitochondria (**Hottenrott** and Neumann, 2010, p. 13).*

The *interval shuttle run test (ISRT)* was developed in 1998 at the Institute of Human Movement Science at Groningen University, Netherlands (Dollemann, 1998), and expanded to a direct performance diagnosis (and also a training aid) through the range of existing interval runs (shuttle run test and the yo-yo tests). Lemmink, Verheijen, and Vissher tested and affirmed it specifically for its soccer-specific validity "[...] for measuring endurance in a more soccer-specific way" (2004, p. 233).

Since 2009, the *interval shuttle run test (ISRT)* has been available in CDformat with a detailed accompanying booklet or its practical implementation in training (Universitair Centrum ProMotion Groningen, 2009).

The players run "[...] at a certain speed in running periods of approx. 30-second increments with 15-second active rest periods (slow cool-down in the 8-m zones)" (Universitair Centrum ProMotion Groningen, 2009). (See fig. 73.) The running back and forth is done at a distance of 20 meters with a fixed protocol for the steadily increasing speed. The running speed specified on the CD by Piepton starts at 6 mph and increases .6 mph every 90 seconds. Once a speed of 8 mph has been reached, the increases go down to .3 mph. The result is determined by the number of completed course sections. The test can be administered in a group setting and can also be specified as a submaximal constant.

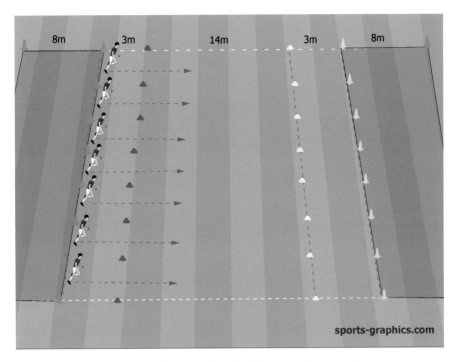

Fig. 73: The Dutch interval shuttle run test (ISRT)—a fitness test for soccer players

Based on the authors' practical experience with the test as an additional testing and training method, the use of the ISRT in advanced youth training is possible, but to date it still lacks testing in the areas of effectiveness and reliability in competitive youth soccer (Hoff, Kähler, and Helgerud, 2006, p. 116-124; Meyer and Fraude, 2006, p. 147-148).[40]

The example given here shall make clear that the inventory of methods and, thereby, the level of knowledge in soccer training and play, in this case, elite-sport oriented, have definitely changed. If, in the 1960s, the running performance of elite soccer players at more than 4,000 meters per game was considered outstanding (Weineck, 2004, p. 24), today's professional soccer players, depending on their position and scope, most often run between 10,000 to 14,000 meters during a competitive game. In the course of a playing season, this brings the pros up to a total of approximately400 kilometers. This is equal to the distance between Cologne, Germany, and Paris, France (Reinhold, 2008). Beyond that, today's demand

---

40 The **Ajax shuttle run** is another soccer-specific test for professional players, which focuses on agility and anaerobic **alactic** capacity (**Tossavainen**, 2004, p. 44).

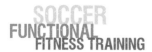

profile in professional soccer is much different, and with respect to space and time, much more intense.

Table 22: Requirement profile in today's pro soccer (ft-Redaktion, 2014, p. 52-53).

Running performance per game based on various criteria			
Teamtactical actions	Individual running performance	Energy parameters	Exertion and recovery
Transitioning to defense:20-30 m in 3-5 seconds	10 to 14 km per game depending on position	Average heart rate between 175-180 BPM	73% of game phases are shorter than 30 seconds
4-6 positional attacks after a counter	Average sprint length: 17 to 22 m	28-30 minutes at 85-90% of maximum heart rate	One-third of all game sequences last approx. 15 seconds
70% of all goals are scored after a quick counter	Total sprint distance depending on position: 300 to 800 m	18-20 minutes at 90-95% of maximum heart rat	52% of rest periods last 15 seconds
70% of all shots on goal come after 2-4 passes	30-55 sprints depending on position	8-12 minutes at 95-100% of maximum heart rate	There is a playing action every 35-43 seconds

As the chart shows, a soccer player must meet the following endurance demands:

- Sustain intermittent exertions for long stretches of time
- Be able to play soccer for a long time in a very intense setting
- Be able to run very fast.

In 2004, Hoff and Helgerud were able to quantify that a team's extra value of approximately 6 ml/kg/min higher maximum oxygen uptake (VO2max) would be about equivalent to a twelfth teammate.[41] Stöggl et al. (2010, p. 43) emphasize that significant relationships exist between VO2max and the completed running distance—the number of sprints and standings at championships.

In light of the studies by Siegle, Geisel, and Lames (2012), the extent to which running distances and running intensities can be viewed as absolute indicators for performance capacity and fatigue in soccer remains debatable. These Munich sports scientists found out that playing position and score have a significant effect (p <

---

41 *For comparison: A professional male soccer player has 55-68 ml/kg/min VO2max.*

0.01) on the running performance of professional soccer players. By contrast, the effect of the opposing team's strength showed an insignificant trend (p = 0.067). These findings show that next to the variable running performance, the many other factors, such as those listed previously and, for example, the importance of the game, motivation, and team tactics, must absolutely be considered and deserve to be the subject of future case studies.

But the results from today's computerized analytic tools provide important information for training design in elite soccer and are generally also available in the pro league youth competitive soccer centers (also see the Adidas mi Coach elite team system).

Next to the data sets on running performances, tactical performance, fatigue, and regeneration,[42] the issues of the training content to be determined and effective methods to improve, in particular, endurance, speed, and power play are of great importance for coaches and instructors. If, as was exemplified at the beginning of this chapter,

"[f]itness training is soccer training, soccer training is fitness training"

(van Lingen, 2001, p. 159)

applies, then

1. there should be empirical evidence that at least does not contradict this as-sertion, and
2. training forms should be introduced that make the effectiveness of the respective training intent obvious.

At least since this statement by former German national team coach, Jürgen Klinsmann, in the **Süddeutsche Zeitung** on September 6, 2004:

"The other's tempo at the European championships was a step above ours—and it won't get any slower in the future"

---

42 *As it is outside the scope of this book, we will not discuss the testing of aerobic and anaerobic endurance capacity in elite soccer here. Instead the authors refer to **Broich, Sperlich, Buitrago, Mathes, and Mester** (2012).*

and Verheijen's publications and lectures in the German-speaking realm (2009a and 2009b), theoretical and practical debates have ensued on whether **high-intensityinterval training (HIIT/HIT)** or **volume-oriented endurance training (HVT/UT)** is more effective in improving endurance performance as well as sprinting and jumping performance in soccer in a shorter period of time.[43]

Moreover, the movement pattern of children and adolescents clearly suggests interval training: low, moderate, and high intensities. Approximately 95% of observed children's activities last no longer than 15 seconds. Studies clearly show that interval exercises are more popular with children than endurance runs (Gahluland Hofmann, 2015, p. 31).

With reference to the exercise standards taken into account in training planning, HIIT and HVT can be tabulated as follows:

3-5x per week	HIIT	HVT
Intensity	90-95% of maximum heart rate	65-75% of maximum heart rate
Duration	15 sec – 4 min	> 45 min
Break	15 sec – 3 min	–
Volume	Approx. 20 min	> 45 min
Frequency	1-3 x per week	3-5x per week

To date there are many empirical findings on the adjustment response and effectiveness of HIIT with respect to endurance capacity as well as its effects on running and takeoff strength in soccer players. The authors will introduce three approaches for the effectiveness and practical use of HIIT and HVT in training (also in comparison and in combination)following

- for men's professional soccer,
- for youth soccer programs in pro soccer clubs, and
- for amateur and semi-pro soccer

---

43   For the sake of completeness, we will at this point refer to threshold training(THR) practiced in endurance sports and polarized training(POL). In THR the exercise intensity is chosen to facilitate lactate threshold training. POL is a blend of HVT and HIIT and is most often practiced at a 70 (HVT): 20 (HIIT): 10 (medium intensity) ratio (**Stöggl** and **Sperlich**, 2014, p. 1-9). Initial study results suggest that in classic endurance sports (running, Nordic skiing, cycling), POL (compared to the previously mentioned types of training) produces the highest increases in VO2max.

without claiming completeness.[44] We will conclude as a last point with the characteristics of the principal physical manifestations and changes brought on by HIIT and HVT.

First approach: Stöggl et al. (2010, p. 43-49) tested the effects of HIIT on running performance and the lasting effects (see table 24) in two studies with a speed group and a control group, using two variations of 12-day HIIT-block (12-14 HIIT-units at 90-95% maximum heart rate; HRmax each) and breaks to be determined:

Table 24: Study results on high-intensity interval (HIIT) and speed training with menstate and national team soccer players

HIIT-block variations	Dribble parcours along a pole cross and 1-on-1 dribble play (15 sec-15 sec)	Speed block	Realistic game-like forms
Exertion	12 units of 15 sec each (64 x 15 sec total/15-sec intervals)	12 units with sprints (all out) for 5-10 m with directional change (alternating sprint)	12-14 units of 4 min playing time each on an approx. 5 x 10 m field per player pair (rule of thumb)
Break	4 units of 15 sec between dribbling and 3 min after each series and 3 units without break	20 sec between sprints and 3 min after each series	3 min at 70-17% HRmax
Repetition	12 units of 4 series of 8 x 15 sec	3 series of 6 sprints	4
Content	Dribble with the ball	Sprints	2-on-2, 3-on-3, 4-on-4, 4-on-2, and games with ball on an open field
Effects	• Increased VO2max with lasting effects • No improvement in sprint performance • Improved performance in alternating sprints with lasting effects	• No change in VO-2max • Increases in tested sprint and alternating sprint performances	• Increased VO2max with lasting effects • No improvements in sprint performance • Increased performance in alternating sprints with lasting effects

---

44 Here we will refer to the *"four-step model"* of the adaptation of fitness-related abilities (Hottenrott and Neumann, 2010, p. 13-19), the *"effects of different recovery protocols after high-intensity interval training"* (Hägele et al., 2009, p. 10-14), and the *"evaluation of running distances in different speed ranges in pro soccer"* (Broich, Brauch, and Mester, 2008, p. 8-12).

The control group that was able to complete normal soccer training for a six-week period used the extensive and intensive interval method for their endurance training. Here the VO2max levels remained unchanged during that period of time.

Of particular importance for soccer practice was the finding that the effects of 4 x 4 minutes or 15 sec-15 sec intervals with soccer-specific training content remained above starting levels throughout the competitive season and the winter break (see above).

Stöggl et al. (2010, p. 48) attribute the positive effects with the use of soccer-specific games on small fields and exertion over time primarily to the greater energy expenditure while running with the ball (approx. 8%) and the use of 2-on-2 forms of play and 2-on-4 inferior number play that proved physically most demanding during the studies. They also determined that spurring on by the coach or instructor was significant in maintaining the necessary intensities (in the study, between 84 and 91%).

To achieve a possible increase in sprint performanceusing the 15 sec-15 sec HIIT variation, Stöggl et al. (2010, p. 49) suggest an increase in intensity toward maximum acceleration at the beginning of this variation.

Stöggl et al. (2010, p. 49) think that an increase in VO2max could be achieved by using speed blocks and by extending the sprint distance up to 40 metersand with uphill sprints, sprints with resistance tools, or jumping variations.

To maintain or even increase VO2max during the competition phase, the authors suggest two HIIT units per week, "[...] whereby the lasting effect of a 2-week HIT-block was still perceptible after 4-7 weeks" (Stöggl et al., 2010, p. 49). When aiming for an improved VO2max and alternating sprint, sprint, and acceleration performance in the training process, the authors suggest the above-mentioned modified 15 sec-15 sec HIIT variation (extend distance up to 40 m and increase number of sprints).

To avoid a negative impact on the effectiveness of the HIITblocks, the authors recommend resting two days after one week of HIIT and three days after completion of the entire HIITblock.

Second approach: In 2010, the German Research Center for Competitive Sports"Momentum" at the German Sport University Cologne and the Institute for Training Science and Sports Informatics at the German Sport University Cologne were able to, under the leadership of Sperlich et al., conduct a comparison study between high-intensity interval training and endurance training with emphasis on volume during the preparatory phase of one of the German Bundesliga premier team's U14 team (see table 25).

Table 25: Training content and breaks of the two interventions for each training unit (TU = training unit; HIT[45] = high-intensity interval training; VT = volume training; B = break) based on Sperlich et al., 2010, p. 122

TE	HITprogram			Volume program		
	Content	Break	Total (min)	Content	Break	Total (min)
1	8 x 1 min 6 x 1 min	1 1	29	6 x 6 min	3	51
2	4 x 4 min	3	29	4 x 12 min fartlek	2	54
3	4 x 4 min	3	29	3 x 30 min fartlek	5	65
4	12 x 30 s sprint, 6 x 2 min	0,5 2	31	4 x 12 min fartlek	2	54
5	4 x 4 min	3	29	3 x 15 min fartlek	3	51
6	5 x 800 m	2,5	25	2 x 25 min fartlek	5	55
7	10 x 400 m	1,5	30	Endurance run (8,9 km)	0	60
8	4,1,1,4,2,4 min	2	26	5 x 10 min fartlek	1	55
9	15 x 200 m	1,5	29	4 x 10 min fartlek	3	69
10	12 x 30 s sprint 6 x 2 min	0,5	31	3 x 15 min fartlek	3	51
11	4 x 4 min	3	29	Endurance run (8,9 km)	0	60
12	4 x 4 min	3	29	2 x 30 min fartlek	5	65
13	4 x 4 min	3	29	2 x 25 min fartlek	5	55
MS ± SD			28,8 ± 1,7			57,3 ± 5,9

---

45 The abbreviations HIT and HIIT are interchangeable in sport science literature. This also applies to VT and HVT.

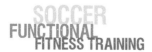
Can a HIIT program training intervention whose volume is reduced by half generate a more positive effect on endurance capacity (VO2max, 1,000-mtime) and vertical leap and sprint times in youth players than the VT program (see table 25). The results can be summarized as follows:

❯ In the HIIT program, players have significantly higher percentages in intensities between 80 to 100% HRmax than in the VT program. Player feedback regarding subjective perceived exertion and the measured arterial lactate concentrations[46] underscore that assertion.

❯ VO2max increased significantly by 7% after HIT and correlated with an improved 1,000-mtime (T1000m) through a significant drop in time with respect to the starting test (on average by -10 seconds after HIT vs. -5 seconds after VT).

❯ Sprint performances improved significantly with HIT and VT for all distances. The research group attributes these effects to the concurrent soccer-specific training.

❯ Vertical leap performance remained unchanged[47] with both training interventions in both groups. This was also true for bodyweight, body fat, and body size. According to the research group, the concurrent soccer-specific training does not appear to contribute to an improved vertical leap. Supplementary strength and coordination training should, therefore, be applied.

❯ With the growing academic obligations and recreational activities of youth players, HIT helps to reduce practice time in the previously mentioned areas without having to accept performance loss and stagnation.

❯ If HIT can be completed three times a week for five weeks, it will result in a significant increase in VO2max and T1000 m.

---

46 To date the formation of lactate in competitive soccer has been viewed primarily in terms of by-product, main factor in muscle fatigue, main factor in acidosis-induced muscle injuries, and overtraining. When taking into account current findings by the German Research Center for Competitive Sport in Cologne, Germany (Momentum), regarding youth players and the elite, lactate, in the future, will also be viewed as fuel (also in the brain), signaling molecule, regulator of tissue adaptation, instigator of collagen synthesis, and additional helper in wound repair.

47 Gahlul and Hofmann (2015, p. 31-35) were able to confirm this missing significant effect in a latest study with 34 Austrian youth soccer players and made the supposition that "[...] clearly the effects of general training are so great, that additional specific training like the applied interval training does not show any obvious effect (in improving vertical leap) (A/N)" (p. 35). They recommend studies with longer training programs. The authors point to the implementation of the content in chapter 14 of this book.

However, in a study on HIT in youth soccer (block periodization[48] of high-intensity interval training),Bieri et al. (2013, p. 307-312) found within the scope of their research design that HIT does not cause an increase in VO2max. They attribute this to the total amount of working time per unit as well as the type of training module. They pose the question of whether "the functional adaptations to high-intensity endurance modulesare at best due to mechanisms of blood regeneration" (p. 312)? Additional intervention studies are pending.

Third approach: To the former German Football Association's fitness trainer and current director of the Dortmund, Germany, pro soccer team, Dr. A. Schlumberger, the physical demand profile of a soccer player is characterized by intermittent exertion with variable, fast, and power-based actions through sprints, jumps, shots, and duels so that during a competitive game a player completes,on average, 1,000 to 14,000 brief actions that change every four to six seconds (Schlumberger, 2006, p. 125).

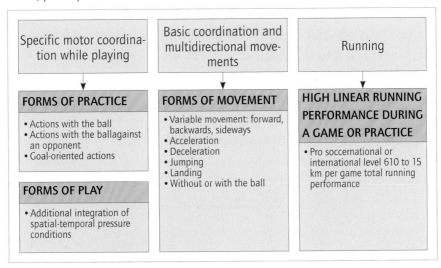

Specific motor coordination while playing	Basic coordination and multidirectional movements	Running
FORMS OF PRACTICE	**FORMS OF MOVEMENT**	**HIGH LINEAR RUNNING PERFORMANCE DURING A GAME OR PRACTICE**
• Actions with the ball • Actions with the ballagainst an opponent • Goal-oriented actions	• Variable movement: forward, backwards, sideways • Acceleration • Deceleration • Jumping • Landing • Without or with the ball	• Pro soccernational or international level 610 to 15 km per game total running performance
FORMS OF PLAY		
• Additional integration of spatial-temporal pressure conditions		

Fig. 74: The basis for soccer-specific fitness training in pro soccer (see Schlumberger, Association of German Soccer Instructors, Westphalia, April 26, 2010

Fitness expert Dr. Schlumberger believes that youth soccer player, in particular,

---

48 *Contrary to classic periodization (Matwejew, 1972 and 1981), the block periodization principle (Issurin, 2003; Issurin and Shakliar, 2002) favors stringing together the development of different motor skills and fitness abilities. It focuses on increasing the workload with the goal of adaptation under consideration of the lingering effects. The concentration of the workload should generate training-related impulses and thereby help to develop primarily sport-specific abilities at a high level of training (Schurr, 2014, p. 102-116).*

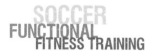

should experience soccer-specific fitness training characterized by economical and skillful movements at a sustained and high-intensity level as a basis for mastering a professional demand profile. This approach is summarized in tabular form in (fig. 74).

To the Dortmund, Germany, fitness expert, as well as the authors, there is a close link between fitness-related abilities and the coordination of soccer-specific movements (see chapters 1 to 7).

He sees the goals of soccer-specific endurance training as follows:

- 90 to 120 minutes optimal performancereadiness for all typical motion sequences in soccer
- Optimal capacity for high-intensity explosive performance in individual actions
- Optimal capacity for repeated high-intensity explosive performance for the duration of the game
- Maintaining the same intensity for a longer period of time
- Achieving a higher intensity within the same period of time
- Good cardiovascular capacity
- Good muscle metabolic function.

Schlumberger (2006) recommends the following content for the three areas of training (see fig. 75):

1. SPECIFIC MOVEMENT COORDINATION—PLAYING

Fig. 75: Forms of play with different emphases within the context of time and space for the

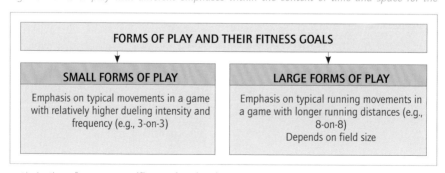

optimization of soccer –specific speed and endurance

He suggests the use of easy to complex training principles, from the consciously to the subconsciously automated,as a key method. Based on Little (2009, p. 67-74), training methodology can be tabulated as follows:

Table 26: Training methodology for the optimization of endurance throughforms of play and as a specific and most effective method for increasing endurance capacity (Stigelbauer, 2010, p. 67)

Training goal/area	% HRmax	Lactate mmol/l	Total time in minutes	Constant repetition	Repetition (R)	Break	Sample form of training
Transition from aerobic to anaerobic	80-90	3-6	30-60	6-30 min	1-8	< 1 min	5-on-5 6-on-6 7-on-7 8-on-8
Maximum oxygen uptake	90-95	6-12	12-35	3-6 min	4-8	0.5:1 to 1:1 break ratio	3-on-3 4-on-4
Anaerobic	> 85	> 10	4-16	20 s- 3 min	2-4 series x 4-8 R	1:1 to 1:4 break ratio	2-on-2 3-on-3 Specified possession

2. BASIC COORDINATION—MULTIDIRECTIONAL MOVEMENTS

For this area Schlumberger (2006) suggests the following workload design, using the example of the preparation period:

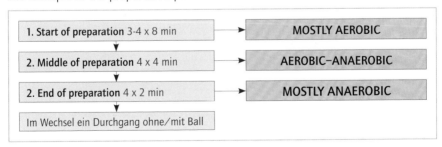

Fig. 76: Workload design for multidirectional movements

---

49 *Dr. Tom Little is currently the director of sports science for the British second division team FC Birmingham.*

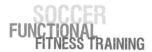

This method can be implemented incisively as practical training through practice exercises and soccer-specific parcours (also to overcome the *ceiling effect*[50]) as preparation and during the season. One example is the dribble parcours as per Hoff et al. (2002).

3. RUNNING

For this area of endurance optimization, the Dortmund pro fitness expert suggests the use of the mostly (aerobic) continuous training method for endurance runs and fartlek. These can be performed extensively and intensively and beyond that also have a regenerative function:

- Compensatory, low-intensity training impulse (focus on immune system)
- Form-stabilizing character ("Watch your form!")
- Optimal adaptations in muscles due to low intensity
- Individualized running training to correct deficiencies
- Mental balance (learning to control by the always keepingthe foot on the gas pedal mindset)

Schlumberger (2010) and Stigelbauer (2010), therefore, definitely argue for the implementation of forms of play at the start of training in amateur and semi-professional soccer, depending on the starting level, as main training methods to improve endurance. In the area of pro soccer, Schlumberger, in particular, suggests the three-part division of soccer-specific endurance training explained previously and emphasizes that particular attention should be paid to the variation training principle combined with the above-threshold training stimulusprinciple of progressive loading.

Characteristics of the important aspects and changes due to HIIT and HVT

HIIT training is currently "the method of choice in soccer fitness training" (Sperlich, 2013, p. 20-22) because it is accompanied by a significant increase in VO2max, does not negatively affect the performance factors speed and takeoff power (and

---

50 *The ceiling effect begins to take place starting with a maximum oxygen uptake of 65 ml/kg/min. Players sometimes show visible signs of this effect during small-field games at practice. They feel unchallenged. Here the player should be sufficiently nurtured and challenged through dribble parcours (Stigelbauer, 2010, p. 63).*

with respect to the modifications in the outlined first approach, can even affect them positively), and requires considerably less training time (compared to HVT).

From a physiological point of view, the change in cardiovascular parameters results in an increased heart size accompanied by a higher heart rate and higher cardiac output (per minute) and due to the increased blood flow, a higher capacity to transport oxygen. This results in faster VO2 kinetics (Stöggl et al., 2010, p. 49). Iaia et al. (2009, p. 291-306) detected increased activity of anaerobic enzymes, membrane transport proteins, and muscle buffer capacity during anaerobic training. These changes resulted in

- a decrease in the inhibiting effects of H+-ions (protons) within the cell,
- an increase in maximum activity of PGC-1 a,[51]
- an increase in proteins that participate in the transport and oxidation of glucose and free fatty acids,
- a densification of the capillaries, and
- an increased training impulse for the fast-twitch muscle fibers.

In table 27, Sperlich, Hoppe, and Haegele (2013, p. 12) summarize the important characteristics of high-intensity interval training (HIIT) and volume-oriented endurance training (HVT) and their sideeffects.

---

51 *PGC-1a is responsible for the mitochondrial biogenesis. Mitochondria are the power stations of the cells—in this case, particularly the muscle cells. It has a positive effect on strength, endurance, and fat burning. We will not elaborate on the significance of AMP-activated protein kinase in connection with the order of training impulses (training planning s. l.) at this time (Schurr, 2014, p. 96).*

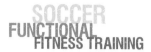

Table 27: The important characteristics of high-intensity interval training (HIIT) and volume-oriented endurance training (HVT)

HIIT	HVT	Commonalities of HIIT and HVT
• Variable exercise form that can be implemented in training in a variety of ways. • Many aerobic and anaerobic, as well as central and peripheral adaptations with little training time. • Provides training stimulus even to endurance-trained athletes. • Improved buffer capacity of skeletal muscles. • The ability to recruit more muscle fibers. • Closer to the soccer-specific demand profile and, therefore, better acclimatization to the workload. • Corresponds to the natural movement behavior of children and adolescents. • No data on long-term effects.	• Large, time-intensive training volume. • Monotonous training. • Loss of speed. • Simpler. • Easier to control. • Better researched.	• Adaptations of aerobic metabolic processes. • Obvious training results after only a short period of time, depending on training status. • Danger of overloading. • Danger of performance stagnation with chronic use. • Improved recovery.

The following is a HIIT pro-and-con summary for competitive youth soccer training:

PRO

❯ There is a direct relationship to soccer: "Fitness abilities in soccer are directly linked to specific movement coordination" (see third approach).

❯ Attractive and motivating fitness training with the ball.

❯ Load increases for adolescents can be controlled.

❯ Prevention of overloading and injuries.

❯ Consideration of scientific principles of progressive loading.

❯ Alternating between maximum explosive power, maximally fast recovery, powerendurance, and retention of quick recovery are highlighted.

❯ Technical and tactical abilities and skills are viewed as key elements in the development of an emerging pro soccer talent.

CONTRA

- Field sizes are too narrow, resulting in exclusively deep play.
- Similar training stimuli do not lead to additional long-term improvement, particularly in acceleration and sprint speed (maximum explosive power).
- An incremental increase of load volume and intensity leads to a performance limit.
- The importance of extensively regenerative endurance runs as a means of recovery and endurance-retention will not be discussed.
- The lack of targeted individualization (including isolated training for the major sport-related motor skill demands) with respect to regulating exertion and regeneration during the wave-like course of the season.
- The exclusive use of soccer-specific exercises results in a speed limit: All three areas, (1) specific movement coordination—playing, (2) basic coordination—multidirectional movements, and (3) running—must be practiced (Schlumberger, 2010).
- No information regarding the use of standardized strength tests.

The pro-and-con arguments show that fitness training in soccer can exist on a continuum between the poles of exclusively standardized performance regulation and the coach's eye and coaching as instruments of subjective training regulation. In between, the experts designate additional hybrid exercises with and without the ball. It would, therefore, be important to the continued development of international youth soccer if sports scientists were able to focus on regulating mechanisms and mechanisms of actions more closely and longterm, particularly in the sensitive areas of advanced and high-performance training.

The interested coach or instructor may, therefore, want to test the presented threeapproachesto contemporary HIIT training in soccer based on his requirement and decision fields and ponder them and closely follow additional research results.[52]

---

52 *Gahlul and Hofmann (2015, p. 31-35) were able to show by means of sprint interval training with adolescent soccer players that a 40-meter sprint interval training already had a significant effect on components of aerobic and anaerobic endurance performance after only 12 training units (two units per week). This training intervention also provided a greater training effect with supplementary extensive endurance running (comparison group) in adolescent players between the ages of 13 and 14.*

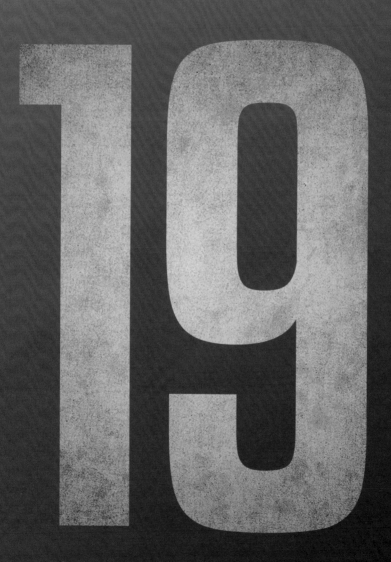

CHAPTER

19

19 EXAMPLES OF SOCCER FITNESS TRAINING DRILLS IN THE CONTEXT OF PERIODIZATION TAKEN FROM MEN'S BUNDESLIGA SOCCER

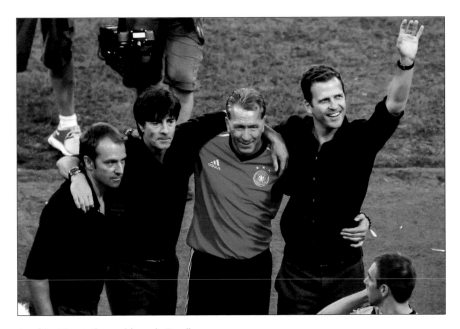

Joachim Löw at the world cup in Brazil

How can soccer fitness training with a German Bundesliga team be implemented on the field within one season? Hereafter, the authors would like to consider this question and present a soccer fitnesstraining program that is already being implemented in one of the Bundesliga men's teams. In doing so, the authors will limit themselves to the descriptions of these exercises and forms of play. Regarding the context of justification, will refer to the exercise executions in chapter 18.

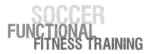

The authors will illustrate examples of the periodization of soccer fitness training as follows:

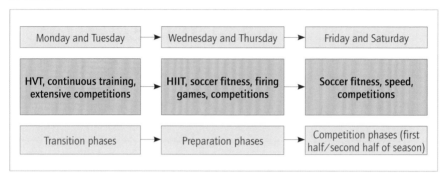

Fig 77: Rough periodization of soccer fitness training for a Bundesliga men's team

SOCCER FITNESS EQUALS SOCCER CONDITIONING!

Intent: Soccer-specific, fitness-based performance factors can be trained at least once a week with HIIT while taking into account the players' existing performance data and current heart rate and lactate concentration measurements combined with the eye of the coach, and can be linked with tactics, technique, creativity, and the joy of playing. Exertion and regeneration times are strictly adhered to and combined with tactics that are generally no longer coached externally during the course of a game. The forms of play are performed in tournament form and linked with penalties for the losers and bonus points for the winners as additional means to increase motivation. The points are transferred to an annual ranking to be posted in the locker room as a Grand Slam chart. One sample drill:

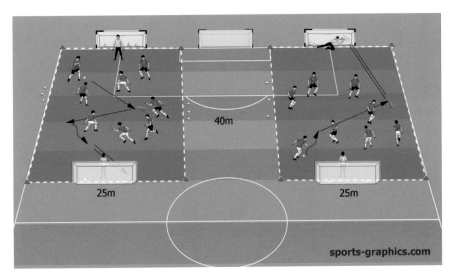

Fig. 78: Power tournaments of 4-on-4 to 6-on-6

ORGANIZATION AND PROGRESSION

- Two fields, 40 x 25 meters,with two goals and two goal players each.
- 4-on-4-tournament.
- Playing time is 12 x 2.5 minutes with 2-minute recovery.
- Keep replacement balls at the ready next to the field and behind the goals to ensure quick continuation of play.

VARIATIONS

- Intensity version: 35 x 20 meter field: 6 x 2 minutes with 3-minute recovery each.
- 5-on-5 on a 50 x 30 meter field: 10 x 3 minutes with 2-minute recovery each.
- High-intensity version: 6-on-6 on a 55 x 35 meter field: 10 x 4 minutes with 3-minute recovery each.
- With three or two goal players, mark another field with mini or youth soccer goals. Only direct goals or doubles count!

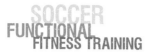

FITNESS TRAINING – FIRING GAMES!

Intent: Within the scope of offensive tactics, the attacker must explode into space before the pass is played (meaning, fire) and run at top speed with the ball that is played into his path. Here the players must solve primarily offensive and defensive 1-on-1 situations in extremely tight spaces and multiple times within a short period of time. Soccer training has proven that in the course of training players are able to implement precise passes even when they are tired. Two examples:

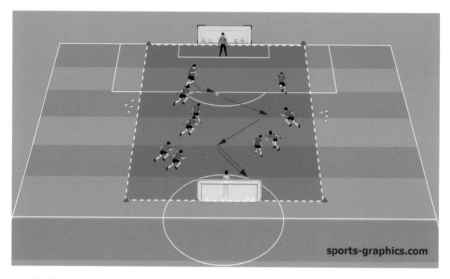

Fig 79: Firing games: 5-on-5 into the running path

ORGANIZATION AND PROGRESSION

- Field is 50 x 30 meters with two goals and goal players.
- 5-on-5: The players are only allowed to play the ball into the running path (not to the body and not to the foot).

COACHING POINTS

- Play risky passes or call for them.
- Operate from positions: don't fire too soon!
- The players must learn that it is also difficult for the opponent to catch up to the ball in the open space.

VARIATIONS

- Larger field: More frequent firing actions and risky passes.
- Pressure of time: Shot on goal within 10, 8, or even 5 seconds.

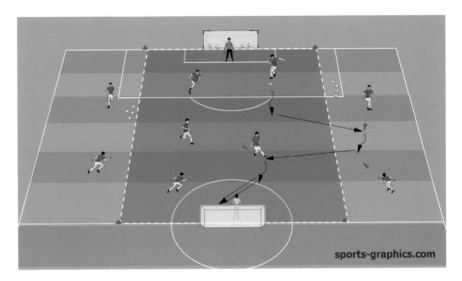

Fig 80: Firing games: 9-on-9 (here without opponent for the sake of better visibilityof field arrangement)

ORGANIZATION AND PROGRESSION

- 9-on-9 on two goals with goal players in one half of a field.
- Mark two outside zones 20 meters wide.
- The pace in the center can drag. The players must fire in the outside zones. Meaning, playing a 1-on-1 either after the pass into the path or with the ball at the foot (feint attacks) are permitted!

COACHING POINTS

- Fire from the center to the outside! Keep sprint pace.
- When under pressure, also play risky balls to the outside.
- Play hard and precise passes.

VARIATIONS

- In the center, play the ball into the pathonly.
- Fire in the center; drag the pace on the outside.

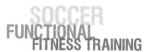
PREPARATION PERIOD – PLAYING WITH HIIT, HVT, ANDBALL AT PRACTICE

Intent: During the preparation phase, the players must work toward the primary goal of increasing endurance capacity (see tables 23 to 27), according to the specifications in chapter 18 as well asthrough HIIT and HVT. In practice, HIIT forms of play can be created by increasing intensity, volume, the number of repetitions, field sizes, the number of games (e.g., 5-on-5 to 7-on-7), adding additional tasks (e.g., all players must move across the centerline), and recovery times. The following are two training examples:

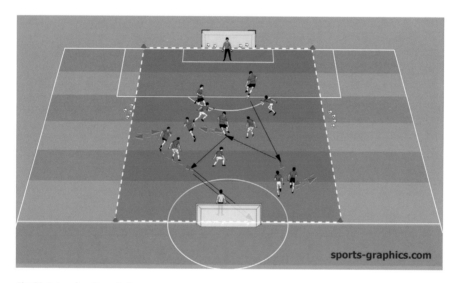

Fig 81: Intensity: 6-on-6 deep

ORGANIZATION AND PROGRESSION
- 6-on-6 with goal players on a field that is 55 x 25 meterswith two goals.
- Playing time is 16 x 2 minutes with 2-minute active recovery.

COACHING POINTS
- Always play deep to increase the tempo.
- Players coach each other.
- The coach only coaches during the final rounds when players are increasingly tired and take breaks.
- Always play from positions.

VARIATIONS

❯ Make the field larger (shift emphasis toward HVT).

❯ Make the field smaller (shift emphasis toward HIIT).

❯ Rule: The opponent is given a penalty kick for every square pass by the team in possession. The pass is taken after the end of the round.

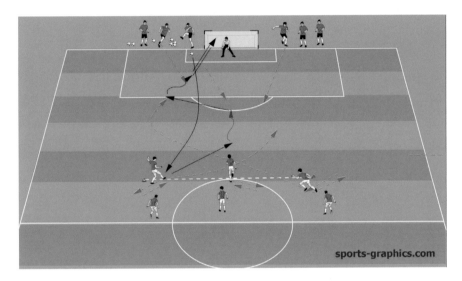

Fig. 82: Intensity: team shot on goal

ORGANIZATION AND PROGRESSION

❯ 6 to 8 defenders with balls stand next to a goal with goal player.

❯ 6 to 8 attacking players face them approximately 30 meters away.

❯ One defender passes to an attacker, after which three players from each group start into the field for 3-on-3.

❯ 8 to 10 repetitions at maximum intensity.

❯ Five-minute recovery with controlled strength exercises.

COACHING POINTS

❯ After the pass, go into the ball.

❯ Both groups immediately look for the 1-on-1.

VARIATION

❯ Increase the number of players.

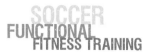

The following are two training examples with a low level of exertion:

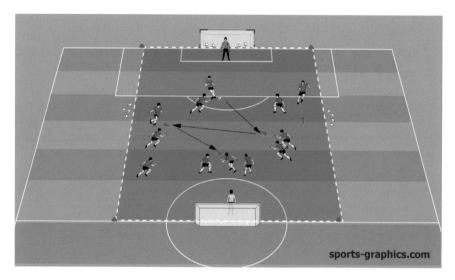

Fig. 83: 6-on-6 with team play as the objective

ORGANIZATION AND PROGRESSION

◈   6-on-6 with goal players on a field that is 55 x 35 meters with two goals.

◈   6 x 3 minutes with three minutes of passive recovery each (e.g., water breaks).

COACHING POINTS

◈   Precise and confidant passing game.

◈   Open body position when receiving and controlling the ball.

◈   Keeping possession.

VARIATIONS

◈   Issuing technical tasks during the rest period.

◈   Sudden death: Ending the round after the first goal.

◈   Interrupting the game when a player makes a careless mistake and then continue play for three minutes.

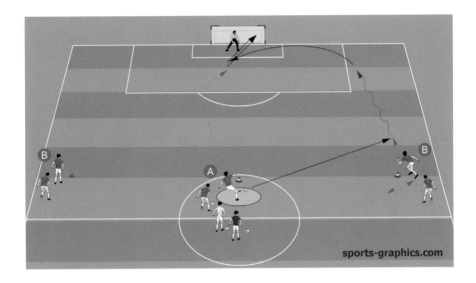

Fig. 84: Double pass sequence

ORGANIZATION AND PROGRESSION

⊘ Form teams of two. Player A stands with the ball 45 meters from a goal with goal player; player B is positioned on the left or right wing without a ball.

⊘ Player A plays a high *double pass* to B, who receives it in the air and controls it, and then crosses it into the path of player A. Player A finishes with a volley.

⊘ Three rounds each (from both sides) with alternating tasks.

⊘ 10 Grand Slam points for the winning team, 8 for the second-place team, and so on.

COACHING POINTS

⊘ Precise and fast *double pass*.

⊘ Settle and control the ball with the first touch.

⊘ Hard cross at a dead run.

VARIATION

⊘ Vary the distances. Guideline for the finish: Goals must be scored with headers.

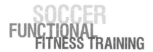
WHO IS THE BEST PLAYER? INDIVIDUAL GRAND SLAM RESULTS!

Intent: Competitions always provide new challenges, especially when they are ongoing. Thus, the authors not only include tournaments or individual forms of play in their own Grand Slam on the practice field, but also a variety of team and individual competitions. These competitions may focus on endurance, technique, or speed.

> *Activate combativeness, ambition, and motivation throughvarious team fitness competitions.*

During team competitions, each player on the winning team gets one point.During individual competitions, points can be staggered: three points for first place, two for second place, and so on. Competitions are particularly well suited to a diverse facilitation and coaching method: sometimes praising, sometimes firmly correcting, sometimes provoking! Next, the authors introduce three forms of competitions:

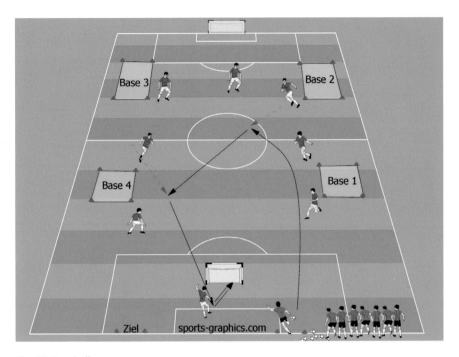

Fig. 85: Baseballsoccer

ORGANIZATION AND PROGRESSION

- Mark four bases on three-quarters of a field and form two teams of eight.

- Team blue stands at the punting spot (circle); team red is fielding.

- Mark a finish line next to or behind the reversed mini goal that is closest to the punting spot.

- The first blue player shoots the resting ball into the field and immediately runs to at least first base.

- Red attempts a combination play in the direction of the mini goal. If the runner is still running at that time, he is burned and must immediately turn back.

- As soon as red has gotten reorganized, the second blue player shoots the ball into the field.

- There can never be two players at one base.

- A home run is worth 10 points. A regular scored run is worth one point.

- Stimulus duration should be 2 x 8 minutes or 4 x 6 minutes.

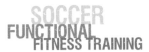

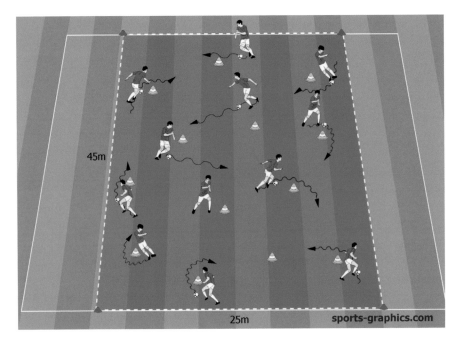

45m

25m

sports-graphics.com

Fig. 86: Chaotic dribbling

ORGANIZATION AND PROGRESSION

- Scatter different color cones around a field that is 45 x 25 meters.
- 12 players perform certain feints while dribbling (e.g., step-over, Beckenbauer 360-turn, drag, Zidane trick, Ronaldo trick, inside roll, lunges).
- To provoke chaos on the field in terms of extreme complexity and pressure of time, the tempo must be kept high at all times.

VARIATION

- Certain feints are assigned to certain color cones (create pressure of variability).

COMPETITIONS

- Collect the different colors.
- Approach 20 cones at a dribble.
- Successive focus on color sequence.
- Combine with taking a shot on four goals, meaning dribble approach to red cone followed by shot on goal 1 (activate distribution ability).

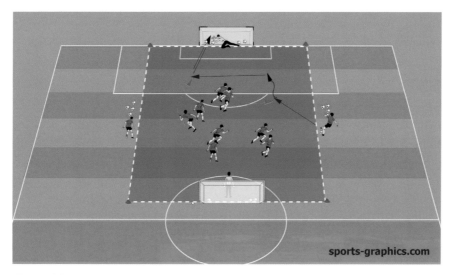

Fig. 87: Firing game

ORGANIZATION AND PROGRESSION

- 4-on-4 with goal players on a field that is 40 x 20 meterswith two goals.
- Coach and assistant coach play the ball into the field from different positions.
- The players promptly take the shot.

COACHING POINTS

- Quickly orient position and immediately adjust to new situations.
- Defender: Make sure the foot is in front of the ball.
- If player chooses to dribble, only do it at a dead run.

VARIATIONS

- Make the field larger and smaller.
- Throw-ins must be high, at hiplevel, and provocative (at the opponent's body or in front of his feet). Or throw in two balls at the same time: The coach calls out which ball should be played (increasing complexity).

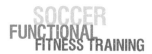
Next and subsequently, the authors will present an example for fitness training in the context of preseason preparation using seven summarized weekly training plans. The first trophy round is the first breakpoint prior to the start of the Bundesliga season:

MAIN OBJECTIVE: DETERMINING THE STARTING BASIS!

Day	Training I 9-10am	Training II 10:30-11:30am	Training III 3-4:30pm
Mon	Field test	Field test	6 x 60 m (60%) form of play
Tue	Internistic training analysis VO2max	Internistic training analysis VO2max	7 x 50 m (70%) 11-on-11/8-on-8 3 x 8 min
Wed	Internistic training analysis VO2max	Internistic training analysis VO2max	8 x 40 m (80%) 11-on-11/8-on-8 3 x 8 min
Thu	Strength/stabilization/ coordination		9 x 30 m (90%) 11-on-11/8-on-8 4 x 13 min
Fri	Strength/stabilization/ coordination	Form of play Young against old	
Sat	Strength/stabilization/ coordination	8 x 40 m (80%) 11-on-11/8-on-8 3 x 13 min	Off
Sun	Off	Off	Off

LEGEND

Green fields ▦ : High-volume training (HVT)

Orange fields : High-intensity training (HIIT)

White fields : Strength/stabilization/coordination

TA: Training analysis

R: Rest period

ST: Soccer tennis

MAIN OBJECTIVE: DAILY STRENGTH, STABILIZATION, COORDINATION,AND SOCCER!

Week of July 5 to July 11

Day	Training I 9-10am	Training II 10:30-11:30am	Training III 3-4:30pm
Mon	Strength/stabilization/ coordination	7 x 50 m (70%) 7-on-7/5-on-5 4 x 3.5 min	Running lanes/crosses/ positioning for the finish
Tue	Strength/stabilization/ coordination	8 x 40 m (80%) 11-on-11/8-on-8 3 x 13.5 min	Open
Wed	Strength/stabilization/ coordination	Firing games 4 x 3.5 min	Running lanes/ positioning/ shot on goal
Thu	Strength/stabilization/ coordination	10 x 20 m 11-on-11/8-on-8 3 x 8 min	Open
Fri	Strength/stabilization/ coordination	GP training 5-on-2/6-on-3 Set pieces/crosses	7pm (45/45) Test game against regional team
Sat	Strength/stabilization/ coordination	GP training Regeneration 10 x 20 m	Open
Sun	Open	Open	7pm (45/45) Test game against regional team

MAIN OBJECTIVE: RAMPING UP BEFORE TRAINING CAMP

Week of July 12 to July 18

Day	Training I 9-10am	Training II 10:30-11:30am	Training III 3-4:30pm
Mon	Strength/stabilization/ coordination	GP training Regeneration	Open
Tue	Open	Open	Open
Wed	Strength/stabilization/ coordination	Positional play/factional play/ shots on goal	8 x 5 m 4-on-4/3-on-3 3 x 3 min (30 sec R)
Thu	Strength/stabilization/ coordination	2 x (6 x 15 m) 7-on-7/5-on-5 4 x 6 min (=9 x 2.5 min)	Open
Fri	Strength/stabilization/ coordination	2 x (8 x 5 m) 4-on-4/3-on-3 3 x 3 min (30 sec R)	Departure for training camp
Sat	Strength/stabilization/ coordination		7pm (60/30) Test game against division 3 team
Sun	Strength/stabilization/ coordination	GP training Regeneration	Open

421

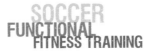

MAIN OBJECTIVE: EAT – SLEEP – TRAIN!

Week of July 19 to July 25

Day	Training I 9-10am	Training II 10:30-11:30am	Training III 3-4:30pm
Mon	Strength/stabilization/ coordination	Running lanes/crosses/shot on goal	8 x 5 m 4-on-4/3-on-3 3 m 3 min (30 sec R)
Tue	Strength/stabilization/ coordination	2 x (6 x 15 m) Firing games 4 x 6 min (= 9 x 2.5)	Running lanes/set pieces/crosses/shot on goal
Wed	Strength/stabilization/ coordination	8 x 5 m Factional play 4-on-4/3-on-3	Test game against division 1 team
Thu	Strength/stabilization/ coordination	Running lanes/set pieces/crosses/shot on goal	2 x (6 x 15 m) 7-on-7/5-on-5 4 x 6.5 min
Fri	Strength/stabilization/ coordination	One touch Firing games 4-on-4/3-on-3	Running lanes/set pieces/crosses/shot on goal
Sat	Strength/stabilization/ coordination	9 x 30 m (90%) 11-on-11/8-on-8 3 x 13.5 min	Open
Sun	Strength/stabilization/ coordination	Open	Test game against division 1 international team

MAIN OBJECTIVE: SOCCER FITNESS

Week of July 26 to August 1

Day	Training I 9-10am	Training II 10:30-11:30am	Training III 3-4:30pm
Mon	Open	Open	Open
Tue	Strength/stabilization/ coordination	11-on-11/8-on-8 3 x 7.5 min	Running lanes/passing lanes/ crosses/shot on goal
Wed	Strength/stabilization/ coordination	Running lanes/set pieces/crosses/shot on goal	Test game against international team
Thu	Strength/stabilization/ coordination	GP training Outside rolls 4-on-4/3-on-3	9 x 30 m (90%) 11-on-11/8-on-8 4 x 11 min
Fri	Strength/stabilization/ coordination	10 x 20 m 11-on-11/8-on-8 3 x 7.5 min	Open
Sat	GP training 5-on-2/6-on-3 Set pieces/crosses	Open	Test game against division 1 international team
Sun	Soccer technique First touch	Season opener	Showtraining

MAIN OBJECTIVE: STARTING TO GET THE ITCH!

Week of August 2 to August 8

Day	Training I 9-10am	Training II 10:30-11:30am	Training III 3-4:30pm
Mon	Open	Open	Open
Tue	Strength/stabilization/ coordination	Positional play	Running lanes/set pieces/crosses/shot on goal
Wed	ST 5-on-2/6-on-3 Set pieces/crosses	Open	7pm (45/45) Test game against a premier league team
Thu	Strength/stabilization/ coordination	Positional play	2 x (8 x 5 m) 2 x (7 x 1.5 m forward/backwards) 4-on-4/3-on-3
Fri	Open	Open	Running lanes/set pieces/crosses/shot on goal
Sat	Strength/stabilization/ coordination	10 x 20 m 11-on-11/8-on-8 3 x 7.5 min	Open
Sun	GP training 5-on-2/6-on-3 Set pieces/crosses	Short-game tournament	Short-game tournament

MAIN OBJECTIVE: ALL EYES ON THE FIRST TROPHY GAME. LOWER VOLUME!

Week of August 9 to August 15

Tag	Training I 9-10am	Training II 10:30-11:30am	Training III 3-4:30pm
Mo.	Strength/stabilization/ coordination	GP training/regeneration 10 x 20 m 4-on-4/3-on-3	Open
Di.	Open	Open	Open
Mi.	Strength/stabilization/ coordination	2 x (8 x 5 m) 4-on-4-tournament	Running lanes/set pieces/ crosses/shot on goal
Do.		10 x 20 m 11-on-11/8-on-8 3 x 7.5 min	
Fr.			11-on-11 Set pieces
Sa.			Firing games Set pieces
So.			National Championships Round 1

> CHAPTER

20

20 CLOSING REMARKS

> *"Everything was just right: the forward movement, the subtle ball control, the finish. The explosion of penalty box denizen [Luis Suárez, FC Barcelona, in a game against Real Madrid (A/N)] with eyes in the back of his head."*

(P. Ingendaay, March 24, 2015,Frankfurter Allgemeine, 70, p. 27)

This book makes no claims of being complete. The chosen subject area is too complex to do so. It is merely intended to make tested and proven tools and present sports scientific findings on the many aspects of their work in the important areas of soccer fitness and athletic training on the practice field available to the many coaches and instructors and support staff with and without trainer certifications or degrees.

To that end, the necessary international sports scientific findings provide conceptual building blocks for the analysis of a coach's training and movement-related questions, but not their solutions. In doing so, the practice would absolutely overwhelm sports science with such a complex subject area as soccer fitness and athletic training. On the contrary, the conveying of general and specific findings in this subject area should primarily help in preventing mistakes in the training process and (well-intentioned) wild actionism through a previous technical analysis and in approaching self-imposed goals in a sustainable and responsible way.

In this respect, the authors tried to include as many old and new areas of soccer fitness training and athletic training as possible without the coach or instructor having to use loads of equipment. Here the associated independent home training of our (hopefully) highly motivated players should not fall from view.

The authors hope that the often secret treasure chest of youth and men's and women's fitness and athletic training has been opened just a little. But coaches and instructors are still responsible for what they can take out of this chest to use with their own team and what they cannot. And during an often arduous and very demanding fitness and athletic training, a positive training and competitive atmosphere is still a top priority.

The players and the team should learn to play better soccer by means of contemporary, well analyzed, and methodologically appealing and variable fitness and athletic training! Training to become a pro instead of high rankings in youth leagues! At this point, success is relative! That's it!

When all the ingredients have been added, the dish should be good! Many of those ingredients can be found in this book. Nevertheless, you, coaches and instructors, determine the hopefully large number of players who continue to develop injuryfree and who may one day wave to us up in the stands of a large stadium or as coaches give us a big hug at the edge of the field.

Moreover, the authors have tried to mark in the text the many sources that were sifted during years of research and transfer them to a list of references at the back of the book. This is not only meant to document legitimate and scientific works, but also to provide the coaches and instructors the opportunity to study this complex subject matter more deeply beyond the content of this book.

At this time, professional soccer, in particular, has, to some extent, reached borderlines of physical and mental stress and strain. This makes long-term, continuous, targeted, coordinated, and joyful fitness and athletic training all the more responsible and important for the players entrusted to us. According to the experts, and based on personal experience, there still are opportunities for positive actions in the future. We hereby present them to you, reader.

Additional sports scientific studies are necessary, particularly in the area of testing and measuring in soccer, to provide coaches and instructors with other important systems of analysis and training aids for the planning and implementation of training with the own team, especially in high-performance training (Granacher, 2015, p. 36-38; Singh, Voigt, and Hohmann, 2015, p. 11-16). Until then, the authors hope that you, reader, will enjoy reading this book. We welcome your tips and suggestions!

Enschede, Cologne, and Leverkusen, Germany, March 2015

> CHAPTER

21

APPENDIX

REFERENCES

⊘ Anderson, K. G. & Behm, D. G. (2005). Trunk muscle activity increases with unstable squat movements. *Can. J. Appl. Physiol., 30*, 33-45.

⊘ Bangsbo, J. (2003). *Fitness training in-soccer. A scientific aproach.* Spring City: Reedswain Publishing.

⊘ Bauersfeld, M. & Voss. G. (1992). *Neue Wege im Schnelligkeitstraining.* Münster: Phillipka Verlag.

⊘ Beck, J. & Bös, K. (1995). *Normwerte motorischer Leistungsfähigkeit − Eine Realanalyse publizierter Testdaten.* Bundesinstitut für Sportwissenschaft: Köln.

⊘ Beck, J., Bös. K., Klaes., L. & Rommel, A. (2006). Entwicklung und Betrieb einer Datenbank zur motorischen Leistungsfähigkeit (SPODAT 2006). In J. Edelmann- Nusser & K. Witte (Hrsg.), *Sport und Informatik* (IX, S. 151-158). Aachen.

⊘ Beilenhoff, A. (2015). Mit CrossFit in die Rückrunde. *fussballtraining, 33* (1 und 2), 18-27.

⊘ Behm, D. & Anderson, K. (2006). The role of instability with resistance training. *Journal Strength Cond. Res. 20,* (3), 716-722.

⊘ Behringer, M., vom Heede., A. & Mester, J. (2009). Krafttraining im Nachwchsleistungssport. In. G Neumann, (Red.), *Talentdiagnose und Talentprognose im Nachwuchsleistungssport* (S. 178). Sportverlag Strauß: Köln.

⊘ Berkmark, A. (1989). Stability of the lumbar spine: A study in mechanical engineering, *Acta Orthop. Scand., 230,* 20-24.

⊘ Bieri, K., Gross, M., Wachsmuth, N., Schmidt, W., Hoppeler, H. & Vogt, M. (2013). HIIT im Nachwuchsfußball − Blockperiodisierung von hochintensivem Intervalltraining. *Deutsche Zeitschrift für Sportmedizin, 64* (10), 307-312.

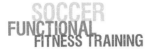
◉ Braun, K. (2014). Bayers Talente geben Gas! *fussballtraining, 32* (3), 14-25.

◉ Broich, H. (2009). *Quantitative Verfahren zur Leistungsdiagnostik im Leistungsfußball.* Unveröffentlichte Dissertation. Deutsche Sporthochschule Köln.

◉ Broich, H. (08.07.2013). *Bayer Leverkusen. Holger Broich: „Besser aufgehoben als bei den Bayern".* http://www.rp-online.de/sport/fussball/bayer-04/holger-broich-besser-aufgehoben-als-bei-den-bayern-aid-1.3520165. Abgerufen am 11.02.2014.

◉ Broich, H., Brauch, S. & Mester, J. (2008). Evaluierung der Laufdistanzen in unterschiedlichen Geschwindigkeitsbereichen im Profifußball. *Leistungssport, 38* (4), 8-12.

◉ Broich, H., Sperlich, B., Buitrago, S., Mathes, S. & Mester, J. (2012). Performance assessment in elite football players: Field level test versus spiroergometry. *Journal of Human Sport & Exercise,* Volume 7, Issue 1, 287-295.

◉ Bruscia, G. (2015). *Handbuch Functional Training.* Aachen: Meyer & Meyer Verlag.

◉ Buckwitz, R. & Stein, R. (2014). Aktuelle Entwicklungen im Kurzsprint der Männer und daraus abgeleitete Schwerpunktsetzungen für das Training. *Leistungssport, 3*, 42-44.

◉ Buffett, W. (04.03.2014). Zitiert in der *Frankfurter Allgemeinen Zeitung, 53*, 25.

◉ Caldwell, B. P. & Peters, D. M. (2009). Seasonal variation in physiological fitness of a semiprofessional soccer team. *Journal of Strength and Conditioning Research, 23* (5), 1370-1377.

◉ Coban, J. (16.03.2015). „Wir dürfen nur schwarze Schuhe tragen". *kicker, 24*, 22.

◉ Coen, B., Urhausen, A., Coen, G. & Kindermann, W. (1998). Der Fußball-Score: Bewertung der körperlichen Fitness. *Deutsche Zeitschrift für Sportmedizin, 49*, 187-192.

◉ Collins, P. (2010). *Kettlebell conditioning – functional strength & power drills.* Aachen: Meyer & Meyer Verlag.

◉ Cometti, G., Mafiuletti., N.-A., Pousson, M., Chatard, J. C. & Maffulli, N. (2001). Isokinetic strength and anaerobic power of elite, subelite and amateur french soccer players. *International Journal of Sports Medicine, 22*, 45-51.

◉ Cronin, J.-B., Hansen, K.-T. (2005). Strength and power predictors of sports speed. *Journal of Strength and Conditioning Research, 19,* 349-357.

- Dante (02.12.2013). Zitiert im *kicker*-Interview mit Zitonni, M., 13.

- Delecluse, C.-D., Van Coppenolle, H., Willems, E., Van Leemputte, M., Diels, R. & Goris, M. (1995). Influence of high-resistance and high-velocity training on sprint performance. *Medicine and Science in Sports and Exercise, 27*, 1203-1209.

- Di Salvo, V., Baron, R., Tschan, H. et al. (2007). Performance charakteristics according to playing position in elite soccer. *Int. J. Sports Med., 28*, 222-227.

- Dollemann, G. (1998). *Interval Sprint & Interval Shuttle Run Test.* Abschlussarbeit des Instituts für Bewegungswissenschaften. Rijksuniversiteit Groningen.

- Durastanti, C. & Durastanti, P. (2008). *Fußballschule für Kinder und Jugendliche – testen-bewerten-gezielt trainieren.* Onli Verlag: Leer.

- Ekstrand, J. (2013). Playing too many matches is negative for both performance and player availability – results from the on-going UEFA Injury Study. *Deutsche Zeitschrift für Sportmedizin, 64*, 1, 5-9.

- Faries, M. D. & Greenwood, M. (2007). Core training: Stabilizing the confusion. *Strength Cond. J., 29* (2), 10-25.

- Feldbusch, E., te Poel, H.-D. & Herborn, D. (2015). *„Faire Zweikampf- und Körperschulung einmal anders!"* DVD. Köln.

- *Frankfurter Allgemeine Zeitung* (4. März 2014). So wurde Warren Buffet reich. *Nr. 53*, S. 25

- Freiwald, J. (2009). *Optimales Dehnen. Sport – Prävention – Rehabilitation.* Balingen: Spitta Verlag.

- Fröhlich, M., Schmidtbleicher, D. & Emrich, E. (2007). Vergleich zwischen zwei und drei Krafttrainingseinheiten pro Woche – ein metaanalytischer Zugang. *Spectrum der Sportwissenschaften, 19* (2), 6-21.

- Fröhlich, M., Gießing, J. & Strack, A. (2009). *Kraft und Krafttraining bei Kindern und Jugendlichen – Schwerpunkt apparatives Krafttraining.* Marburg: Tectum.

- Fröhner, G. & Tronick, W. (2007). Prophylaxe von Verletzungen und Fehlbelastungsfolgen durch Belastbarkeitssicherung im Nachwuchsleistungssport. *Leistungssport, 37* (1), 11-17.

- ft-Redaktion (2014). Fitness mit Ball à la Suisse. *fussballtraining, 32* (6+7), 52-63.

- Fuchs, R. K., Bauer, J. J., Snow, C. M. (2001). Jumping improves hip and lumbar spine bone mass in prepubescent children: A randomized controlled trial. *J. Bone Miner Res.2001 Jan:16* (1): 148-156.

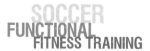

❂ Gahlul, S. A. & Hofmann, P. (2015). Sprint-Intervalltraining bei jugendlichen Fußballern. *Leistungssport, 2,* 31-35.

❂ Gambetta, V. (2007). *Athletic developement: The art & scienceof functional sportsconditioning.* Human Kinetics.

❂ Geisler, I. (2013). Ropetraining – vielfältig und belastungsintensiv. *fussballtraining, 31* (6+7), 48-55.

❂ Geisler, I. (2014). Kleine Rolle, große Wirkung! Leistungsreserve Faszien-Training. *fussballtraining, 32* (6+7), 72-78.

❂ Granacher, U. (2015). WVL-Projekt Krafttraining im Nachwuchs Leistungssport (Kings-Studie). *Leistungssport, 2,* 36-38.

❂ Greier, K. & Riechelmann. H. (2012). Ballspielverletzungen im Schulsport und Möglichkeiten der Prävention. *Deutsche Zeitschrift für Sportmedizin, 2012: 63,* 168-172.

❂ Grosser, M. (1991). *Schnelligkeitstraining.* BLV Sportwissen: München.

❂ Güllich, A. (1996). *Schnellkraftleistungen im unmittelbaren Anschluss an maximale und submaximale Krafteinsätze.* Sport und Buch Strauß GmbH: Köln.

❂ Gustedt, C. (2013). Zum Einfluss von Rumpfkraft und -stabilität auf die sportliche Leistungsfähigkeit. *Leistungssport, 43* (2), 11-15.

❂ Hägele, M., Wahl, P., Sperlich, B. & Mester, J. (2009). Aktiv oder passiv – der Effekt unterschiedlicher Erholungsprotokolle nach hochintensivem Intervall-Training (HIT). *Leistungssport, 39* (6), 10-14.

❂ Hartmann, O. (25.09.2014). WM unter der Lupe. *kicker, 40* (80), 88-89.

❂ Hirtz, P. (1997). *Bewegungskoordination und sportliche Leistung integrativ betrachtet.* Hamburg: Czwalina.

❂ Hodges, P. W. & Richardson, C. A. (1996). Inefficient muskular stabilization of the lumbar spine associated with low back pain. A motor control evaluation of transversus abdominis. *Spine, 21,* 2640-2650.

❂ Höhner, O. (2012). Herausforderungen an die Talentforchung im Fußball. *Deutsche Zeitschrift für Sportmedizin 63* (9), 270-271.

❂ Hoff, J. (2005). Training and testing physical capacities for elite soccer players. *Journal of Sports Sciences, 23* (6), 573-82.

❂ Hoff, J., Wisløff, U., Engen, L., Kemi, O. & Helgerud, J. (2002). Soccer specific aerobic endurance training. *British Journal of Sports Medicine, 36,* 218-221.

Hoff, J. & Helgerud, J. (2004). Endurance and strength training for soccer players: Physiological considerations. *Sports Medicine, 34* (3), 165-180.

Hoff, J., Kähler, N. & Helgerud, J. (2006). Training sowie Ausdauer und Krafttests von professionellen Fußball-Spielern. *Deutsche Zeitschrift für Sportmedizin, 57* (5), 116-124.

Hoff, J. & Helgerud, J. (2004). Endurance and strength training for soccer players. Physiological considerations. *Sports Medicine, 34*, 165-180.

Hohmann, A. (2001). Leistungsdiagostische Kriterien sportlichen Talents. *Leistungssport, 31*, 14-22.

Hohmann, A., Lames, M. & Letzelter, M. (2002). *Einführung in die Trainingswissenschaft.* Wiebelsheim: Limpert Verlag.

Hossner, E. J. (1995). *Module der Motorik.* Schorndorf: Hofmann.

Hottenrott, H. & Neumann, G. (2010). Ist das Superkompensationsmodell noch aktuell? *Leistungssport, 40* (2), 13-19.

Hotze, N. (2014). „Hier schießt niemand aus der Hüfte". Borussia. *Das Mitgliedermagazin, 81,* 62-65.

Hyballa, P. & te Poel, H.-D. (2015). *Modernes Passspiel.* Aachen: Meyer & Meyer. 3. Auflage.

Hyballa, P. & te Poel, H.-D. (2013). *Mythos niederländischer Nachwuchsfußball.* Aachen: Meyer & Meyer. 2. Auflage.

Iaia, F. M., Rampinini, E. & Bangsbo, J. (2009). High-intensity training in football. *International Journal Sports Physiology Performance, 4*, 291-306.

Ingendaay, P. (24.03.2015). Zerfallene Schönheit: Suárez erledigt Real. *Frankfurter Allgemeine Zeitung, 70,* 27.

Issurin, V. B. (2013). Training transfer: Scientific background and insights for practical application. *Sports Medicine, 43* (8), 675-697.

Issurin, W. (2003). Aspekte der kurzfristigen Planung im Konzept der Blockstruktur. *Leistungssport, 5,* 41-44.

Issurin, W. & Shkliar, W. (2002). Zur Konzeption der Blockstruktur im Training von Hochklassifizierten. *Leistungssport, 6,* 42-45.

Javanovic, M., Sporis, G., Omrcen, D. & Fiorenti, F. (2011). Effects of speed, agility and quickness training method on power performance in elite soccer players. *Journal of Strength and Conditioning Research, 25* (5), 1285-1292.

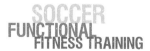
- Kibler, WB., Press, J. & Sciascia, A. (2006). The role of core stability in athletic function. *Sports Med., 36* (3), 189-198.

- Killing, W. (2008). *Leistungsreserve Springen.* Philippka Sportverlag: Münster.

- Kindermann, W., Gabriel, H., Coen, B. & Urhausen, A. (1993). Sportmedizinische Leistungsdiagnostik im Fußball. *Deutsche Zeitschrift für Sportmedizin, 44* (6), 232-244.

- Kleinöder, H. (2004). Kraft: Diagnostik und Training, Praxis- und Laborverfahren, isometrische, isokinetische und dynamische Diagnostik, Trainingsumsetzungen. In *Sport ist Spitze. Landesprogramm Talentsuche und Talentförderung. Ruhrolympiade* (58-65). Marl.

- Kleinöder, H. (2009). Krafttraining in den Spielsportarten. In G. Neumann (Red.*), Talentdiagnose und Talentprognose im Nachwuchsleistungssport* (179-180). Köln: Sportverlag Strauß.

- Kollath, E. (1996). *Bewegungsanalyse in den Sportspielen: Kinematisch-dynamische Untersuchungen mit Empfehlungen für die Praxis.* Köln: Sport und Buch Strauss.

- Kollath, E., Merheim, G., Braunleder, A. & Kleinöder, H. (2006). Sprintschnelligkeit von jugendlichen Leistungs-Fußballspielern. *Leistungssport, 36* (3), 25-28

- Kollath, E. & Buschmann, J. (2010). *Fußball Stabilisationstraining.* Meyer & Meyer Verlag: Aachen.

- König, S., Memmert, D. & Moosmann, K. (Hgg.) (2012). *Das große Limpert-Buch der Sportspiele. Regeln, Technik und Spielformen von Mannschafts- und Rückschlagspielen.* Wiebelsheim: Limpert Verlag.

- Kotzamanidis, C., Chatzopoulos, D., Michailidis, C., Papaiakovou, G. & Patikas, D. (2005). The effect of a combined high-intensity strength and speed training program on the running and jumping ability of soccer players. *J Strength Cond Res., 19* (2), 369-375.

- Kröger, C. & Roth, K. (2014). *Koordinationsschulung im Kindes- und Jugendalter.* Hofmann-Verlag: Schorndorf.

- Lames, M., Augste, C., Dreckmann, C., Görsdorf, K. & Schimanski, M. (2008). Der „Relative Age Effect" (RAE): neue Hausaufgaben für den Sport. *Leistungssport, 38* (6), 4-9.

- La Torre, A., Vernillo, G., Rodigari, A., Maggioni, M. & Merati, G. (2007). Explosive strength in female 11-on-11 versus 7-on-7 soccer players. *Sport Science and Health, 2,* 80-84.

- Lehmann, F. (1993). Schnelligkeitstraining im Sprint. *Leichtathletiktraining, 4* (5/6), 9-16.

- Lemmink, K. A. P. M., Verheijen, R. & Visscher, C. (2004). The discriminative power of the Interval Shuttle Run Test and the Maximal Multistage Shuttle Run Test for playing level of soccer. *Journal of Sports Medicine and Physical Fitness, 44* (3), 233-239.

- Little, T. (2014). Der Fitness-Trainer muss den Fußball kennen! *fussballtraining, 32* (1+2), 62-64.

- Little, T. (2009). Optimizing the use of soccer drills for physiological development. *Strength and Conditioning Journal, 31* (3), 67-74.

- Lockie, R. G., Murphy, A. J., Schultz, A. B., Knight, T. J. & Janse de Jonge, X. A. K. (2012). The effects of different speed training protocols on sprint acceleration kinematics and muscle strength and power in field sport athletes. *Journal of Strength and Conditioning Research, 26* (6), 1539-1550.

- Lopez-Segovia, M., Palao Andrés, J. M. & Gonzáles-Badillo, J. J. (2010). Effect of 4 month of training on aerobic power, strength and acceleration in two under-19 soccer teams. *Journal of Strength and Conditioning Research, 24* (10), 2705-2714.

- Lottermann, St., Laudenklos, P. & Friedrich, A. (2003). Techniktraining – mehr als reine Ballarbeit. Ein Testverfahren zur Diagnostik technisch-koordinativer Fähigkeiten. *fussballtraining, 4,* 6-15.

- Löw, J. (22.12.2014). „Es gibt keinen Fluch des Titels. Dieser WM-Titel steht." *kicker, 104,* 8-13.

- Lüchtenberg, D. & Görgner, C. (2010). *Perfektes Krafttraining mit der SAK-Methode.* Stuttgart: Pietsch Verlag.

- Lühnenschloss, D. & Diercks, B. (2005). *Schnelligkeit.* Schorndorf: Verlag Karl Hofmann.

- Lutz, H. (2010). *Besser Fußball spielen mit Life Kinetik®.* München: BLV Buchverlag.

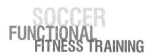
◉ Magnusson, P., Simonsen, E., Henriksorenson, P. & Kjaer, M. (1996). A mechanism for altered flexibility in human skeletal muscle. *Journal Physiology, 497* (1), 291-298.

◉ Mandelbaum, B. R., Silvers, H. J., Watanabe, D. S., Knarr, J. F., Thomas, S. D., Griffin, L. Y., Kirkendall, D. T & Garrett, W. Jr. (2005). Effectiveness of a neuromuscular and proprioceptive training program in preventing anterior cruciate ligament injuries in female athletes: 2-year follow up. *Am J Sports Med, 33*, 1003-1010. doi:10.1177/0363546504272261.

◉ Mann, R. (1999). Biomechanische Grundlagen des Kurzsprints. *Leichtathletiktraining, 10* (2), 24-31.

◉ Martin, D., Nicolaus, J., Ostrowski, Ch. & Rost, K., (1999). *Handbuch Kinder- und Jugendtraining.* Schorndorf: Hofmann.

◉ Masuda, K., Kikuhara, N., Demura, S., Katsuta, S. & Yamanaka, K. (2005). Relationship between muscle strength in various isokinetic movements and kick performance among soccer players. *J Sports Med Phys Fitness, 45* (1), 44-52.

◉ Matwejew, L. P. (1972). *Periodisierung des sportlichen Trainings.* Berlin: Bartels & Wernitz.

◉ Matwejew, L. P. (1981). *Grundlagen des sportlichen Trainings.* Berlin.

◉ McGill, S. M., Childs, A. & Liebenson, C. (1999). Endurance time for low back stabilization exercises: Clinical targets for testing and training from a normal database. *Arch. Phys. Med Rehabil., 80*, 941-944.

◉ McGill, S. M. (2002). *Low back disorders. Evidence-based prevention and rehabilitation.* Champain (IL): Human-Kinetics.

◉ McKeon, P. O., Ingersoll, C. D., Kerrigan, D. C., Saliba, E., Benett, B. C. & Hertel J. (2008). Balance training improves functional and postural contol in those with chronic ankle instability. *Med Sci Sports Exerc, 40*, 1810-1819. doi:10.1249/MSS.0b013e31817e0f92.

◉ Meier, H. (2011). Möglichkeiten des sensomotorischen Trainings – Slacklinetraining. *Leistungssport, 41* (5), 42-45.

◉ Memmert, D. & Roth, K. (2003). Individualtaktische Leistungsdiagnostik im Sportspiel. *Spectrum der Sportwissenschaften, 15*, 44-70.

◉ Memmert, D., Strauss, B. & Theweleit, D. (2013). Der Fußball – die Wahrheit. München: Süddeutsche Zeitung Edition.

⚫ Mester, J. & Kleinöder, H. (2008). Kraftstatus und Trainierbarkeit im Nachwuchsbereich. In Schriftenreihe des Bundesinstituts für Sportwissenschaft (Hrsg.) *Krafttraining im Nachwuchsleistungssport.* (S. 27-48). Leipziger Verlagsanstalt: Leipzig.

⚫ Meyer, T., Coen, B., Urhausen, A., Wilking, P., Honorio, S. & Kindermann, W. (2005). Konditionelles Profil jugendlicher Fußballspieler. *Deutsche Zeitschrift für Sportmedizin, 56*, 1, 20-25.

⚫ Meyer, T. & Faude, O. (2006). Feldtests im Fußball. *Deutsche Zeitschrift für Sportmedizin, 57* (5), 147-148.

⚫ Miller, F. P., Vandome, A. F. & McBrewster, J. (Hrsg.). (2010). *Pyramide Des Besoins de Maslow.* Alphascript Publishing.

⚫ Müller-Wolfarth, H.-W. & Schmidtlein, O. (2007). *Besser Trainieren!* München: Zabert Sandmann Verlag.

⚫ Myer, G. D., Paterno, M. V., Ford, K. R. & Hewett, T. E. (2008). Neuromuscular training techniques to target deficits before return to sport after anterior cruciate ligament reconstruction. *Journal Strength Cond Res., 22* (3), 987-1014.

⚫ Myer, G. D., Brent, J. L., Ford, K. R. & Hewett, T. E. (2008). A pilot study to determine the effect of trunk and hip focussed neuromuscular training on hip and knee isokinetic strength. *British Journal of Sports Medicine, 42*, 614-619.

⚫ Naul, R., Hoffmann, D., Nupponen, H. & Telama, R. (2003). PISA-Schock auch im Schulsport? Wie fit sind finnische und deutsche Jugendliche? *Sportunterricht, 52*, (5), 137-141.

⚫ Neumaier, A. & Mechling, H. (1999). *Koordinatives Anforderungsprofil und Koordinationstraining.* Köln: Sport & Buch Strauß.

⚫ Neumann, G. (2009). *Talentdiagnose und Talentprognose im Nachwuchsleistungssport.* 2. BISP-Symposium: Theorie trifft Praxis. Bonn.

⚫ Newman, M. A., Tarpenning, K. M. & Marino, F. E. (2004). Relationships between isokinetic knee strength, single-sprint performance, and repeated-sprint ability in football players. *J Strength Cond Res., 18*, (4), 867-72.

⚫ Ohlert, J. & Kleinert, J. (2014). Entwicklungsaufgaben jugendlicher Elite-Handballerinnen und -Handballer. *Zeitschrift für Sportpsychologie, 21*, (4), 161-172.

⚫ Oltmanns, K. (2009). *Gymnastik für das Aufwärmen.* Münster: Philippka Sportverlag.

- Oltmanns, K. (2009b). *Sprungkraft systematisch aufbauen.* Münster: Philippka Sportverlag.
- Paradisis, G. P & Cooke, C. B (1996). The effects of combined uphill downhill training on sprint performance. *Journal Sport Science. 14,* 96.
- Patra, S. (2011). Mit Power in die Rückrunde. *Fußballtraining, 29* (1+2), 70-83.
- Pfaff, E. (2013). „Das Wichtigste war und ist, dass wir immer auf Augenhöhe agiert haben." Interview mit Holger Geschwindner in *Leistungssport, 3,* 49-53.
- Pfeifer, K., Bös., Tittlbach, S., Stoll, O. & Woll, A. (2001). Motorische Funktionstests. In Bös, K. (Hrsg.), *Handbuch Motorische Tests.* (209-251). Hogrefe-Verlag: Göttingen.
- Pieper, S. & Kleinöder, H. (2006). *Testverfahren zur Messung von Schnelligkeits- und Kraftfähigkeiten der Beine.* o. O. und Verlag.
- Raab, M. (2000). *SMART. Techniken des Taktiktrainings – Taktiken des Techniktrainings.* Köln: Sport und Buch Strauß.
- Redenius-Heber, J. & Weist, G. (2005). *Diagnostik von Defiziten in den koordinativen Komponenten elementarer Fertigkeiten im Sportspiel Fußball.* Unveröffentlichte Diplomarbeit, Paderborn, Universität.
- Reinhold, T. (2008). *Leistungsdiagnostik im Fußball.* Saarbrücken: VDM Verlag Dr. Müller.
- Richardson, C., Jull, G., Hodges, P. & Hides, J. (1999). *Therapeutic exercise for spinal segmental stabilization in low back pain: Scientific basis and clinical approach.* Edinburgh (NY): Churchill Livingstone.
- Riegler, L. & Stöggl, T. (2014). Effizienzuntersuchung eines sechswöchigen Rumpfkrafttrainings. Vergleich von Sling-Training und konventionellem Rumpfkrafttraining. *Leistungssport, 44* (1), 20-23.
- Ronnestad, B. R., Kvamme, N. H., Sunde, A. & Raastad, T. (2008). Short-term effects of strength and plyometric training on sprint and jump performance in professional soccer players. *Journal of Strength and Conditioning Research, 22* (3), 773-780.
- Ronnestad, B. R., Nymark, B. S. & Raastad, T. (2011). Effects of in-season strength maintenance training frequency in professional soccer players. *Journal of Strength and Conditioning Research, 25* (10), 2653-2660.
- Roth, K. (1996). *Techniktraining im Spitzensport.* Köln, Sport und Buch Strauß.

- Roth, K. (2005). Koordinationstraining. In A. Hohmann, M. Kolb & K. Roth (Hrsg.). *Handbuch Sportspiel* (327-334). Schorndorf: Verlag Karl Hofmann,
- Roth, K. (2005). Techniktraining. In A. Hohmann, M. Kolb & K. Roth (Hrsg.). *Handbuch Sportspiel* (335-341). Schorndorf: Verlag Karl Hofmann,
- Roth, K., Memmert, D. & Schubert, R. (2006). *Ballschule Wurfspiele.* Schorndorf: Hofmann.
- Roth, K. & Kröger, Ch. (2011). *Ballschule. Ein ABC für Spielanfänger.* Schorndorf: Hofmann-Verlag.
- Roth, K., Damm, T., Pieper, M. & Roth, C. (2013). *Ballschule in der Primarstufe.* Schorndorf: Hofmann.
- Roth, K., Damm, T., Memmert, D. & Althoff, T. (2014). *Ballschule Torschussspiele.* Schorndorf: Hofmann.
- Roth, K., Roth, C. & Hegar, U. (2014). *Mini-Ballschule. Das ABC des Spielens für Klein- und Vorschulkinder.* Schorndorf: Hofmann-Verlag.
- Rowland, T. W. (2004). *Children's exercise physiology.* Champaign: Human Kinetics.
- Sadres, E., Eliakim, A., Constantini, N., Lidor, R. & Falk, B. (2001). The effect of long-term resistance training on anthropometric measures, muscle strength, and self concept in pre-pubertal boys. *Ped Exerc Sci 13*, 357-372.
- Sahin, H. (09.03.2015). „Die Defensive ist meine Stärke". *kicker, 22,* 18-19.
- Sander, A., Keiner, M., Wirth, K. & Schmidtbleicher, D. (2012). Entwicklung von Sprintleistungen durch ein Krafttraining im Nachwuchsleistungssport Fußball. *Spectrum der Sportwissenschaften, 24* (2), 28-46.
- Sander, A., Keiner, M., Wirth, K. & Schmidtbleicher, D. (2013). Leistungsunterschiede im schnellen und langsamen Dehnungs-Verkürzungszyklus bei Fußballspielern in Abhängigkeit von Alter und Spielklasse. *Leistungssport, 43* (4), 24-28.
- Schiffers, M. (2014). Die Körpermitte mit dem Deuserband stark machen! Trainingsprogramm zur Verbesserung der Rumpfkraft. *fussballtraining, 32* (1+2), 66-75.
- Schurr, S. (2014). *Trainingsplanung und -steuerung im Ausdauersport. Block- und klassische Periodisierung als alternative Planungsmodelle?!* Norderstedt: Books on Demand.

- Schlumberger, A. (2006). Sprint- und Sprungkrafttraining bei Fußballspielern. *Deutsche Zeitschrift für Sportmedizin, 57* (5), 125-131.

- Schlumberger, A. (2010). *Fitnesstraining bei den DFB-Junioren.* PPP-Vortrag im Rahmen der BDFL-Fortbildung der Verbandsgruppe Westfalen vom 26. April in der Sport-Centrum Kaiserau.

- Schmidtbleicher, D. (1984). *Sportliches Krafttraining und motorische Grundlagenforschung.* Heidelberg.

- Schmitt, H. (2013). Prävention und Therapie typischer Verletzungen und Überlastungsbeschwerden bei männlichen Fußballspielern. *Deutsche Zeitschrift für Sportmedizin, 64,* (1), 18-27.

- Schöllhorn, W. I., Sechelmann, M., Trockel, M, & Westers, R. (2006). Nie das Richtige trainieren, um richtig zu spielen. *Leistungssport, 5,* 13-17.

- Schöllhorn, W. I. (2003). *Eine Sprint- und Laufschule für alle Sportarten.* Aachen: Meyer & Meyer Verlag.

- Schöllhorn, W. I., Hegen, P. & Eckhoff, A. (2014). Differenzielles Lernen und andere motorische Lerntheorien. *Spektrum der Sportwissenschaften, 2,* 35-55.

- Siegle, M., Geisel, M. & Lames, M. (2012). Zur Aussagekraft von Positions- und Geschwindigkeitsdaten im Fußball. *Deutsche Zeitschrift für Sportmedizin, 63,* 278-282.

- Silvestre, R., Kraemer, W. J., West, C., Judelson, D. A., Spiering, B. A., Vingren, J. L., Hatfiled, D. L., Anderson, J. M. & Maresh, C. M. (2006). Body composition and physical performance during a national collegiate athetic association division I men's soccer season. *Journal of Strength and Conditioning Research, 20* (4), 962-970.

- Singh, A., Voigt, L. & Hohmann, A. (2015). Konzepte erfolgreichen Nachwuchstrainings (KerN). *Leistungssport, 2,* 11-16

- Souid, K. (2011). *Zum Einfluss von Muskelkraft, Beweglichkeit und Schnelligkeit sowie neuromuskulärer Koordinationsfähigkeit auf die Verletzungsanfälligkeit des Gelenkes. – Grundlagen zu präventiven Maßnahmen im Elitefußball.* Dissertation am Institut für Biomechanik und Orthopädie der Deutschen Sporthochschule Köln.

- Sperlich, B. (2013). HIT – derzeit DIE Methode im Fußball-Fintnesstraining. *fussballtraining, 31* (6+7), 20-22.

- Sperlich, B., Hoppe, M. W. & Haegele, M. (2013). Ausdauertraining – Dauermethode versus intensive Intervallmethode im Fußball. *Deutsche Zeitschrift für Sportmedizin, 64* (1), 10-17.

- Sperlich, B., Eder, F., Broich, H., Krüger, M., Zinner, C. & Mester J. (2010). Vergleich von intensivem Intervalltraining vs. umfangsbetontem Ausdauertraining in der Vorbereitungsphase im U14-Fussball. *Schweizerische Zeitschrift für „Sportmedizin und Sporttraumatologie", 58* (4), 120-124.

- Steinhöfer, D. (2003). *Grundlagen des Athletiktrainings.* Münster: Philippka-Sportverlag.

- Steinhöfer, D. (2008). *Athletiktraining im Sportspiel.* Münster: Philippka-Sportverlag.

- Steinhöfer, D. (2014). Langhanteltraining im Leistungssport ist kein Gewichtheben. *Leistungssport, 44* (1), 14-19.

- Stigelbauer, R. (2010). *Spezielles Ausdauertraining im Fußballsport. High Intensity Training in Form von Kleinfeldspielen zur Entwicklung der maximalen Sauerstoffaufnahme.* VDM Verlag Dr. Müller AG & Co. KG: Saarbrücken.

- Stöggl, T., Stiegelbauer, R., Sageder, T. und Müller, E. (2010). Hochintensives Intervall-(HIT) und Schnelligkeitstraining im Fußball. *Leistungssport, 40* (5), 43-49.

- Stöggl, T. & Sperlich, B. (2014). Polarized training has greater impact on key endurance variables than treshold, high intensity, or high volume training. *www.frontiersin.org*, Volume 5, Article *33*, 1-9. Abgerufen am 12. September 2014.

- Swiss Olympic (2003). Manual Swiss Olympic. *Qualitätsentwicklung Sportmed Swiss Olympic, Leistungsdiagnostik Kraft, Version 2.0.*

- Stolen, T., Chamari, K., Castagna, C. & Wisloff, U. (2005). Physiology of soccer. An update. *Journal of Sports Medicine, 35,* 501-536.

- Szymanski, B. (1997). *Techniktraining in den Sportspielen – bewegungszentriert oder situationsbezogen?* Hamburg, Czwalina.

- Taube, W. (2012). Neurophysiological adaptions in response to balance training. *German Journal of Sports Medicine, 63* (9), 163-167.

- te Poel, H.-D./Herborn, D. (2015). Faire Zweikampf- und Körperschulung. Fußball – einmal (ganz) anders! In: *sportunterricht. Lehrhilfen für den Sportunterricht*, 64. Jg., H.11, 9-14.

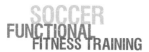
❂ te Poel, H.-D. & Hyballa, P. (2015). *Modernes Passspiel international.* Aachen: Meyer & Meyer Verlag.

❂ te Poel, H.-D. & Hyballa, P. (2011). Wenn das Fußballtalent im Mathematikunterricht an den Doppelpass denkt! Wechselwirkungen zwischen Schule und Fußball im Leben eines zukünftigen Nationalspielers. *Leistungssport, 4*, 33-38.

❂ te Poel, H.-D. & Eisfeld, H. (1987a). Verbesserung der Schnelligkeit im Fußball. 1. Teil: Vorbemerkungen und Trainingseinheit zur Verbesserung der Koordination (ohne Ball). *fußballtraining, 5* (11), 3-10.

❂ te Poel, H.-D. & Eisfeld, H. (1987b). Verbesserung der Schnelligkeit im Fußball. 2. Teil: Vorbemerkungen und zwei Trainingseinheiten zur (1) Verbesserung des Start- und Reaktionsvermögens (ohne Ball) und zum (2) Schnelligkeitstraining mit Ball. *fußballtraining, 5* (12), 31-35.

❂ te Poel, H.-D. & Eisfeld, H. (1988). Verbesserung der Schnelligkeit im Fußball. 3. Teil: Allgemeine Vorbemerkungen zum Krafttraining im Fußball und Trainingseinheit zur Verbesserung der Sprint-/Startkraft. *fußballtraining, 6* (1), 21-28.

❂ Timmermanns, W. (2010). *Injury prevention and strength training in soccer by mobility and flexibility.* DVD: Act2Prevent.

❂ Tossavainen, M. (2004). *Testing athletic performance in team and power sports.* Oulu.

❂ Ullrich, B., Alexander, N., Stening, J., Felder, H. & Hökelmann, A. (2014). Veränderungen der Ermüdungswiderstandsfähigkeit der Rumpfmuskulatur als Folge einer 10-wöchigen kraftausdauerorientierten Trainingsintervention bei Nachwuchsathleten. *Leistungssport, 44* (3), 12-24.

❂ Ülsmann, T. (2012). *Konditionstraining für Fußballer.* Meyer & Meyer Verlag: Aachen.

❂ Universitair Centrum Pro Motion Groningen. (2009). *Intervall Shuttle Run Test (ISRT).* Leer.

❂ Valdez, N. (23.02.2015). „Schaaf ist jetzt ein anderer Mensch". *kicker, 18*, 78-79.

❂ van Lingen, B. & Pauw, V. (1999/2000). Das Trainieren von Jugendfußballern. In R. Verheijen (Red.), *Handbuch Fussballkondition* (226-236). Leer: bfp Versand Anton Lindemann.

❂ van Lingen, B. (2001). *Coachen van jeugdvoetballers.* Zeist: KNVB.

- Verheijen, R. (Red.). (1999/2000). *Handbuch Fußballkondition.* Leer: bfp Versand Anton Lindemann.
- Verheijen, R. (2009a). Warum die Russen so fit waren. *fußballtraining, 27* (1+2), 26-32.
- Verheijen, R. (2009b). Trainieren Sie traditionell oder richtig? *fußballtraining, 27* (10), 6-14.
- Verstegen, M. & Williams, P. (2006). *Core-Performance.* München: Riva Verlag.
- Voss, G. & Witt, M. (1998). Bewegungsgesteuerte Neuromuskuläre Stimulation – BNS. *Leistungssport, 28* (1), 43-47.
- Voss, G., Witt, M. & Werthner, R. (2007). *Herausforderung Schnelligkeitstraining.* Aachen: Meyer & Meyer-Verlag.
- Wegmann, G. (2012). *Dehnen und Kräftigen für Fußballspieler. 51 Schulungsfilme zur Optimierung der körperlichen Voraussetzungen.* DVD: ohne Verlag und Ort.
- Weineck, J. (2004). *Optimales Fußballtraining.* Balingen: Spitta-Verlag.
- Weineck, J. (2007). *Optimales Training.* Balingen: Spitta-Verlag.
- Weineck, J., Memmert, D. & Uhing, M. (2012). *Optimales Koordinationstraining im Fußball. Sportwissenschaftliche Grundlagen und ihre praktische Umsetzung.* Balingen: Spitta-Verlag.
- Williams, A. M., Lee, D. & Reilly, T. (2000). Talent identification and development in soccer. *Journal of Sport Science, 18,* 657-667.
- Wienecke, E. (2007). *FIT Gewinnt. Ran an die Leistungsreserven von Fußballern.* Münster: philippka.
- Wild, K. (3.11.2014). Mission Messi. *Kicker, 90,* 8-11.
- Wirth, A., Bob, A., Müller, S. & Schmidtbleicher, D. (2011). Vergleich unterschiedlicher Belastungsintensitäten zur Steigerung der Schnellkraft. *Leistungssport, 41* (1), 36-42.
- Wirth, A., Schlumberger, A., Zawieja, M. & Hartmann, H. (2012). *Krafttraining im Leistungssport. Theoretische und praktische Grundlagen für Trainer und Athleten.* Köln: Sportverlag Strauß.
- Wisloff, U., Castagna, C., Helgerud, J., Jones, R. & Hoff, J. (2004). Strong correlation of maximal squat strength with sprint performance and vertical jump height in elite soccer players. *British Journal of Sports Medicine, 38,* 285-288.

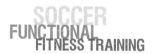
❯ Wollny, R. (2002). *Motorische Entwicklung in der Lebensspanne.* Schorndorf: Hofmann.

❯ Young, W.-B., McDowell M.-H. & Scarlett B.-J. (2001). Specificity of sprint and agility training methods. *Journal of Strength and Conditioning Research, 15,* 315-319.

❯ Young, W.-B., James, R. & Montgomery, I. (2002). Is muscle power related to running speed with changes of direction? *Journal of Sports Medicine and Physical Fitness, 42,* 282-288.

❯ Zafeiridis, A., Saraslanidis, P., Manou, V., Ioakimidis, P., Dipla, K. & Kellis, S. (2005) The effects of resisted sled-pulling sprint training on acceleration and maximum speed performance. *Journal Sports Medicine Physical Fitness. 45,* 284-290.

❯ Zatciorsky, V. M. (1996). *Krafttraining. Praxis und Wissenschaft.* Aachen: Meyer & Meyer.

❯ Zawieja, M. (2008). *Leistungsreserve Hanteltraining. Handbuch des Gewichthebens für alle Sportarten.* Münster: Philippka Sportverlag.

❯ Zawieja, M. & Oltmanns, K. (2011). *Kinder lernen Krafttraining.* Münster: Philippka Sportverlag.

❯ Zitouni, M. (13.10.2014). Hart am Limit. *kicker (84),* 12-13.

CREDITS

Cover design:	Claudia Sakyi
Cover photos:	©Imago/Sportfotodienst
Editing:	Elizabeth Evans
Composition and graphics:	Claudia Sakyi
Interior layout:	Claudia Sakyi
Jacket photos:	©Thinkstock/iStock/ingram_publishing
Interior photos:	Theo Temmink, Harry Dost, and Hans-Dieter te Poel
	©picture-alliance/dpa: p. 41, 77, 81, 87, 119, 135, 325, 374, 375

Players from the FC Twente/Heracles youth team

In chapter 16: Eddie Pasveer doing professional goal player training with the Vario band.

In chapter 16.2.6: Eduard Feldbusch (Bachelor of Sport scientist/German Sports University Cologne) doing athletic individual training with the kettlebell.

In chapter 16.2.7: Julius Duchscherer (NC State Wolfpack and member of the All-Freshman-Team) doing individual *athletic training* with the Sling Trainer.

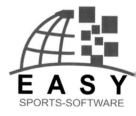